O A C L

OXFORD AMERICAN CARDIOLOGY LIBRARY

Heart Failure: A Practical Guide for Diagnosis and Management

Stuart D. Katz, MD

Helen L. and Martin S. Kimmel Professor of Advanced
   Cardiac Therapeutics
Leon H. Charney Division of Cardiology
New York University School of Medicine
New York, New York

Series Editor

Ragavendra R. Baliga, MD, MBA, FACC, FRCP

Director of Cardiovascular Medicine
The Ohio State University Medical Center
Columbus, Ohio

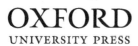

OXFORD
UNIVERSITY PRESS

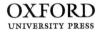

OXFORD
UNIVERSITY PRESS

Oxford University Press is a department of the University of Oxford.
It furthers the University's objective of excellence in research, scholarship,
and education by publishing worldwide.

Oxford   New York
Auckland   Cape Town   Dar es Salaam   Hong Kong   Karachi
Kuala Lumpur   Madrid   Melbourne   Mexico City   Nairobi
New Delhi   Shanghai   Taipei   Toronto

With offices in
Argentina   Austria   Brazil   Chile   Czech Republic   France   Greece
Guatemala   Hungary   Italy   Japan   Poland   Portugal   Singapore
South Korea   Switzerland   Thailand   Turkey   Ukraine   Vietnam

Oxford is a registered trademark of Oxford University Press
in the UK and certain other countries.

Published in the United States of America by
Oxford University Press
198 Madison Avenue, New York, NY 10016

© Oxford University Press 2013

Library of Congress Cataloging-in-Publication Data
Katz, Stuart D., author.
Heart failure : a practical guide for diagnosis and management / Stuart Katz.
    p. ; cm.—(Oxford American cardiology library)
Includes bibliographical references and index.
Summary: "Clinical practice consensus guidelines for management of heart failure are available
from the American Heart Association/American College of Cardiology, Heart Failure Society of
America, Canadian Cardiovascular Society, and European Society of Cardiology. The guidelines
from these organizations, based on evidence from clinical trials and expert agreement, are largely
concordant and provide useful information for practitioners. Yet, the organization of the guidelines
may confound efforts by a practitioner to determine which specific intervention, or combination
of interventions, are most appropriate for an individual patient. As part of the Oxford American
Cardiology Library, Heart Failure utilizes the staging of heart failure proposed by the ACC/AHA
guidelines as a framework to develop a systematic approach for diagnosis and treatment across a
broad spectrum of clinical presentations. Each chapter addresses a different stage in the progression
of heart failure and provides a patient-centered description of the appropriate diagnostic and
treatment options for that setting. Each chapter also incorporates discussion of the diagnosis and
treatment options for both low ejection fraction heart failure patients and preserved ejection
fraction heart failure patients, of which the latter group comprises at least 50% of all heart failure
cases in clinical practice. Heart Failure restructures the information in the clinical guidelines to a
format that is more accessible and clinically useful to practitioners"—Provided by publisher.
ISBN 978–0–19–991708–2 (pbk. : alk. paper)
I. Title.   II. Series: Oxford American cardiology library.
[DNLM: 1. Heart Failure—diagnosis.   2. Heart Failure—therapy. WG 370]
RC685.C53
616.1′29—dc23   2013013465

9 8 7 6 5 4 3 2 1
Printed in the United States of America
on acid-free paper

Contents

Preface

As a cardiologist with subspecialty interest in heart failure for over 20 years, I have been fortunate to witness the development of new pharmacological and device therapies that have dramatically improved the quality of life and survival in patients with chronic heart failure. Implementation of these new therapies into clinical practice has been slower than anticipated, and fewer than half of eligible patients are actually receiving all the therapies known to improve survival in heart failure. Most heart failure patients are diagnosed and treated in primary care practices. Accordingly, there is a need to increase knowledge of heart failure pathophysiology, clinical assessment, and management strategies among primary care providers in order to increase the appropriate utilization of proven treatment modalities in this population.

Clinical practice consensus guidelines for management of heart failure are available from national and international cardiovascular disease scientific societies (listed in the Appendix). The guidelines from these organizations, based on evidence from clinical trials and expert consensus, are largely concordant and provide useful information for practitioners. However, the organization of the guidelines, based on categorizing the scientific hierarchy of the existing evidence in support of various therapeutic interventions, may hinder efforts by a practitioner to determine which specific intervention, or combination of interventions, is most appropriate for an individual patient.

The writing of this book was undertaken with the goal of providing a concise and practical guide for busy practitioners who are engaged in the clinical care of patients with chronic heart failure. This book is not meant to duplicate the content of existing guidelines, but rather to provide a framework for practical implementation of the guideline recommendations in clinical practice. I have chosen to utilize the staging of heart failure proposed by the American College of Cardiology/American Heart Association guidelines as a framework to develop a structured approach for the diagnosis and treatment of heart failure across a broad spectrum of clinical presentations.

Much of the content is based on my clinical experience and practice, but relevant articles from the medical literature are cited throughout the book in support of my recommendations. I have strived to provide the rationale for my personal approach to the management of patients with heart failure, but acknowledge that there exists a great deal of variability in practice among heart failure subspecialists, and in many cases, more than one valid approach to a problem. The practice of medicine remains an art, not a cookbook recipe. The content of the book is not intended to dictate a single approach to management, but rather to provide relevant information to assist clinical decision making in practice settings.

My hope is that this book will provide a valuable resource for all practitioners involved in the care of patients with heart failure, either as a brief overview of the field, or as a concise reference for specific problems encountered in clinical practice. No single text can hope to cover every possible scenario encountered in clinical practice. I am hopeful that the proposed structured approach will bring some clarity to the complex decision-making process required for this management of heart failure and will be useful for practical optimization of care in this patient population.

Stuart Katz

Acknowledgments

This book could not have been written without the cooperation of the thousands of patients with chronic heart failure who have allowed me to participate in their care over the last three decades. Their shared life experiences have provided the basis for my understanding of the pathophysiology and treatment of heart failure. My hope is that the content of this book will be used to improve the lives of patients suffering from this disease.

I would also like to thank my wife and children for their enduring love and support through my many long hours of patient care, scientific meetings, and book and manuscript preparation. Their presence in my life is a continuing source of inspiration, without which this book would not have been possible.

Lastly, I am indebted to my mentors and role models Dr. Thierry LeJemtel, Dr. Edmund Sonnenblick, and Dr. Milton Packer, who not only introduced me to the basic principles of heart failure pathophysiology and management, but also taught the art of creative reflection that has greatly enriched my clinical work, research, and writing.

Stuart Katz

Chapter 1

Definition of Heart Failure

Key Points

- Heart failure is best defined as a clinical syndrome, a recognizable cluster of typical signs and symptoms related to venous congestion and reduced organ perfusion.
- Typical signs and symptoms of the clinical syndrome heart failure have limited sensitivity and specificity.
- Heart failure diagnosis should be classified by left-ventricular ejection fraction (reduced vs. preserved ejection fraction).

"Heart failure" can be defined based on a description of its pathophysiology, or based on a description of the clinical syndrome associated with its pathophysiology.

Heart failure is a pathophysiological state in which the heart is unable to pump sufficient blood to meet the metabolic needs of the body tissues at normal cardiac filling pressures. While heart failure is usually associated with abnormal cardiac structure and function, this definition of heart failure encompasses a diverse array of conditions, including some conditions in which the heart may be structurally and functionally normal (such as high output heart failure states due to severe anemia or arteriovenous shunts). As further discussed, in Chapter 3, heart failure pathophysiology is best considered as a form of circulatory failure, with its clinical manifestations attributable to primary defects in cardiac structure and function and associated secondary changes in peripheral circulations and skeletal muscle metabolism that impair peripheral oxygen utilization.

From a clinical perspective, heart failure can best be defined as a clinical syndrome, a recognizable cluster of typical signs and symptoms related to venous congestion and reduced organ perfusion (Table 1.1). This syndromic definition of heart failure is useful for clinical practice, but it must be applied with the following caveats in mind:

- Most of the signs and symptoms of heart failure are non-specific.
- Many of the signs and symptoms of heart failure have low sensitivity.
- Atypical signs and symptoms are common.

Signs and symptoms of heart failure are listed in Table 1.1. The clinical implications of the above caveats are discussed in Chapters 8 through 10. Specific criteria for the clinical diagnosis of heart failure based on signs and symptoms

Table 1.1 Signs and Symptoms of Heart Failure

	Related to Venous Congestion	Related to Reduced Organ Perfusion
Symptoms	Dyspnea on exertion	Dyspnea on exertion
	Cough	Fatigue
	Paroxysmal nocturnal dyspnea	Lethargy
	Orthopnea	Generalized weakness
	Abdominal swelling	Impaired concentration
	Abdominal fullness	Depression/dysthymia
	Abdominal pain	Agitation/anxiety
	Lower extremity swelling	Anorexia
Physical Findings	Elevated jugular venous pressure	Tachycardia
	Rales	Hypotension
	Decreased breath sounds	Narrow pulse pressure
	Basilar dullness to percussion	Thready pulse
	S3 gallop	Pulsus alternans
	Hepatomegaly	Cool extremities
	Hepatojugular reflux	
	Ascites	
	Lower extremity edema	
Diagnostic Testing Findings	Pulmonary vascular congestion on chest X-ray	Azotemia
	Pulmonary edema on chest X-ray	Lactic acidosis
	Pleural effusion on chest X-ray	
	Abnormal liver function tests	
	Dilutional anemia	
	Hyponatremia	
	Elevation of brain natriuretic peptide levels	

have been established (but not rigorously validated against gold standard hemo-dynamic measurements) for the Framingham study population (Table 1.2).[1,2] Although not used in clinical practice settings, familiarity with these criteria is useful for interpretation of population-based published studies of heart failure (in which Framingham criteria are often used to define the population) and serves as a model for the application of the syndromic definition of heart failure in clinical practice.

Heart failure is usually classified with reference to a descriptor of left-ventric-ular function associated with the clinical manifestations of disease. Throughout this book, I will use the terms *heart failure with reduced ejection fraction* (usu-ally defined as "left-ventricular ejection fraction <40%") and *heart failure with preserved ejection fraction* (usually defined as "left-ventricular ejection fraction ≥40%"). These descriptors are useful for clinical decision-making, as most heart failure clinical trials have been conducted in populations defined in part by the left-ventricular ejection fraction. The selected cut-off value for left-ventricular ejection fraction of 40% is a compromise between the accepted lower limits of normal left-ventricular ejection fraction (typically 50%–55% by most imaging

Table 1.2 Framingham Criteria for Diagnosis of Heart Failure

Diagnosis of heart failure requires the simultaneous presence of at least two major criteria, or one major criterion in conjunction with two minor criteria.

Major Criteria:

Paroxysmal nocturnal dyspnea

Neck vein distention

Rales

Radiographic cardiomegaly (increasing heart size on chest radiography)

Acute pulmonary edema

S3 gallop

Increased central venous pressure (>16 cm H_2O at right atrium)

Hepatojugular reflux

Minor Criteria:

Bilateral ankle edema

Nocturnal cough

Dyspnea on ordinary exertion

Hepatomegaly

Pleural effusion

Decrease in vital capacity by one-third from maximum recorded

Tachycardia (heart rate >120 beats/min.)

Major or Minor Criteria:

Weight loss >4.5 kg in five days in response to treatment.

Minor criteria are acceptable only if they are not attributable to another medical condition (such as pulmonary hypertension, chronic lung disease, cirrhosis, ascites, or the nephrotic syndrome).

modalities), and the entry criteria for clinical trials of patients with reduced ejection fraction (typically <35%). Billing codes use an older terminology of *heart failure with systolic dysfunction* (reduced ejection fractions) vs. *heart failure with diastolic dysfunction* (preserved ejection fraction). Diastolic function cannot be reliably assessed with the imaging techniques routinely available in clinical practice, so the term "diastolic dysfunction" in clinical practice is inferred from the evidence of a heart failure syndrome in the setting of a preserved ejection fraction. Abnormalities in left-ventricular ejection fraction and indices of left-ventricular diastolic function may exist without a clinical heart failure syndrome (further discussed in Chapter 7).

Hypertrophic cardiomyopathy falls broadly under the category of heart failure with preserved ejection fraction, but this group of familial diseases, most often attributable to specific gene mutations in the contractile proteins, requires specialized evaluation and treatment that in many cases is distinct from that of other forms of heart failure with preserved ejection fraction. Consensus guidelines for management of this population have been recently published.[3] In most cases, patients with this form of heart failure should be referred to specialized treatment centers. Diagnosis and treatment of this subgroup of patients with heart failure with preserved ejection fraction will not be further considered in this book.

Other etiological descriptors are often attached to heart failure (*ischemic, non-ischemic, alcoholic,* etc.), but these terms may be misleading because they imply a causal relationship between the descriptor and the heart failure syndrome that may or may not exist. *Heart failure with co-morbid ischemic heart disease* (or other condition) is a more precise terminology that will be used throughout this book. Temporal descriptors (*acute, subacute, chronic*) are also frequently used without specifically assigned time frames to define these terms. In this book, *acute* will refer to syndromes of sudden onset (minutes to hours) without prodromal symptoms; *subacute* will refer to syndromes of gradual onset (hours to weeks); and *chronic* will refer to long-standing disease processes (months to years). *Right-sided heart failure* vs. *left-sided heart failure* are descriptive terms used to indicate a predominance of congestive signs and/ or symptoms in the systemic venous circulation vs. pulmonary venous circulation, respectively. Since the most common cause of systemic venous congestion (right-sided heart failure) is pulmonary venous congestion (left-sided heart failure), these conditions generally do not occur as distinct entities. Finally, older literature often refers to *forward* vs. *backward* heart failure in discussion of pathophysiology. The modern view of the pathophysiology of heart failure is consistent with the forward failure theory as discussed in detail in Chapter 3.

References

1. Marantz PR, Tobin JN, Wassertheil-Smoller S, et al. The relationship between left-ventricular systolic function and congestive heart failure diagnosed by clinical criteria. *Circulation*. 1988;77:607–612.

2. McKee PA, Castelli WP, McNamara PM, Kannel WB. The natural history of congestive heart failure: the Framingham study. *N Engl J Med*. 1971;285:1441–1446.

3. Gersh BJ, Maron BJ, Bonow RO, et al. 2011 ACCF/AHA guideline for the diagnosis and treatment of hypertrophic cardiomyopathy: a report of the American College of Cardiology Foundation/American Heart Association task force on practice guidelines. *Circulation*. 2011;124:e783–831.

Chapter 2

Risk Factors and Natural History of Heart Failure

Key Points

- Heart failure is a common form of heart disease affecting 5–6 million people in the United States.
- Risk factors for heart failure include history of myocardial infarction, hypertension, and increasing age.
- Clinical heart failure is most often preceded by a clinically silent, asymptomatic phase of heart disease.
- Symptomatic heart failure is associated with high risk of hospitalization and death.
- Risk of adverse clinical outcomes in patients with heart failure with reduced ejection fraction and in patients with heart failure with preserved ejection fraction are comparable.

Heart failure is a common cardiac disease affecting between 5–6 million persons in the United States. Most cases of heart failure are associated with the presence of other chronic cardiovascular diseases that lead to cardiac injury (most often in the form of myocardial infarction) or increased cardiac workload (most often in the form of hypertension). Hypertension is the most common risk factor for heart failure. Hypertension is thought to be causally associated with development of heart failure, but definitive studies of a causal link are lacking. Myocardial infarction has been causally linked to the development of heart failure in experimental studies and is associated with a lifelong increased risk of heart failure after an index event.

Other common risk factors are chronic medical diseases commonly associated with hypertension and myocardial infarction (obesity, diabetes mellitus, smoking; population-attributable risk estimates from different populations are provided in Table 2.1).[1–4] Heart failure occurs in men at a younger age and is more often associated with systolic dysfunction (left-ventricular ejection fraction <40%) than it is in women.[5]

In most instances, heart failure is an indolent, progressive disease with a long pre-clinical period of asymptomatic cardiac disease lasting years or even decades. Accordingly, the first presentation of even mild symptoms of heart failure is usually an indication of advanced, long-standing, underlying heart disease.

Table 2.1 **Estimates of population-attributable risk (%) for development of heart failure for common risk factors. The population-attributable risk estimates the proportion of the population that would be free of heart failure if the risk factor were eliminated from the population. Accordingly, if the risk factors listed in this table were eliminated from a given population, the cumulative effect would be a reduction in heart failure by >50%**

	Framingham[1] N = 5143	NHANES[2] N = 13643	CHS[3] N = 5625	Olmstead County[4] N = 1924
Hypertension	Men 39/Women 59	10	13	20
Coronary artery disease	Men 34/Women 13	62	13	20
Obesity	–	8	–	12
Diabetes mellitus	Men 6/Women 12	3	8.3	12
Smoking	–	17	–	14

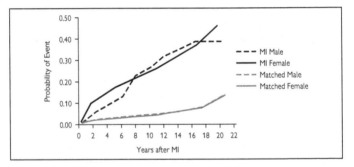

Figure 2.1 Estimate of risk of heart failure over time by gender in patients with history of myocardial infarction and matched controls (from Cupples LA, D'Agostino RB, Some risk factors related to the annual incidence of cardiovascular disease and death using pooled repeated biennial measurements: Framingham Heart Study, 30-year follow-up. In: Kannel WB, Wolf PA, Garrison RJ, eds. *The Framingham Study: An Epidemiological Investigation of Cardiovascular Disease*, section 34, DHHS publication No. (NIH) 87–2703, Washington, DC, US Government Printing Office, 1987; pp. 12–19). The subjects with history of myocardial infarction have greater risk of heart failure when compared with controls. The risk of heart failure continues to rise steadily even >10 years after the index myocardial infarction.

The natural history of heart failure with reduced ejection fraction has been best characterized in patients with a history of myocardial infarction. There is a lifelong increase in the risk of developing heart failure after myocardial infarction for both men and women, when compared with controls without prior myocardial infarction (Figure 2.1). The incidence reported in studies varies according to the clinical features of the index myocardial infarction (infarct size, left-ventricular ejection fraction, and presence of heart failure at the time of the infarction), and the medical therapy received after the infarction. In clinical practice, it is not uncommon to see the first manifestations of heart failure five to ten years after an index myocardial infarction.

The natural history of heart failure with preserved ejection fraction has not been well characterized. While long-standing hypertension is thought to be an important factor in disease progression, a substantial percentage of patients with heart failure with preserved ejection fraction do not have hypertension. The cause of heart failure in non-hypertensive patients is difficult to determine. Infiltrative cardiomyopathies such as senile cardiac amyloidosis (wild-type transthyretin amyloidosis) may be a common cause of heart failure with preserved ejection fraction in elderly subjects without hypertension. Left-ventricular ejection fraction decreases over time in this population, so some patients will eventually be reclassified as having heart failure with reduced ejection fraction.

The natural history of heart failure has also been characterized for patients with some forms of symptomatic valvular heart disease. The reader is referred to existing consensus guidelines for details of the clinical management of valvular heart disease.[6] In most instances, the presence of symptomatic heart failure thought to be attributable to primary valvular heart disease represents a state of advanced heart disease for which surgical intervention is often recommended.

Other less common causes of heart failure due to various primary or secondary cardiomyopathies have varying natural histories specific to each underlying disease state. Younger age, the absence of coronary artery disease, higher left-ventricular ejection fractions, and well-preserved functional capacity are typically associated with a more benign course of disease. Progressive limitation of functional capacity and symptomatic ventricular arrhythmias are associated with worse prognoses.

Since even mild clinical manifestations of symptomatic heart failure are markers of advanced underlying heart disease, clinical diagnosis of heart failure, regardless of the underlying cause, is associated with greatly increased risk of hospitalization and death when compared with control patients without heart failure. Hospitalization for heart failure is an important sentinel event marking an extreme increase in risk of re-hospitalization and death after discharge. Heart failure is the most common primary diagnosis for acute care hospitalization in the Medicare population, but rates of hospitalization for heart failure have been slowly declining over the past decade. Risk of death is comparably increased for patients with heart failure and low ejection fraction and patients with heart failure and preserved ejection fraction.

The Seattle Heart Failure Model is a validated prognostic score that can be useful to assess prognosis and the impact of therapeutic interventions in ambulatory patients with heart failure with reduced ejection fraction.[7] This model is based on clinical and laboratory characteristics that are routinely available in most patients (accessible on the World Wide Web at URL http://depts.washington.edu/shfm/). Predicted survival is provided based on the values entered into the model and the presence or absence of guideline-recommended therapies. Calculation of the prognostic score can assist in clinical decision-making for referral to heart failure subspecialists for evaluation of advanced therapies (heart transplantation and mechanical circulatory support), for assessment of the potential benefits of an implantable defibrillator and/or cardiac resynchronization pacing device, and for clinical decision-making in discussions of end-of-life care.

References

1. Levy D, Larson MG, Vasan RS, Kannel WB, Ho KK. The progression from hypertension to congestive heart failure. *JAMA*. 1996;275:1557–1562.

2. He J, Ogden LG, Bazzano LA, Vupputuri S, Loria C, Whelton PK. Risk factors for congestive heart failure in U.S. men and women: National Health and Nutrition Examination Survery I (NHANES I) epidemiologic follow-up study. *Arch Intern Med*. 2001;161:996–1002.

3. Gottdiener JS, Arnold AM, Aurigemma GP, et al. Predictors of congestive heart failure in the elderly: the cardiovascular health study. *J Am Coll Cardiol*. 2000;35:1628–1637.

4. Dunlay SM, Weston SA, Jacobsen SJ, Roger VL. Risk factors for heart failure: a population-based case-control study. *Am J Med*. 2009;122:1023–1028.

5. Chen YT, Vaccarino V, Williams CS, Butler J, Berkman LF, Krumholz HM. Risk factors for heart failure in the elderly: a prospective community-based study. *Am J Med*. 1999;106:605–612.

6. Bonow RO, Carabello BA, Kanu C, et al. ACC/AHA 2006 Guidelines for the Management of Patients with Valvular Heart Disease: A Report of the American College of Cardiology/American Heart Association Task Force on Practice Guidelines (writing committee to revise the 1998 guidelines for the management of patients with valvular heart disease): Developed in collaboration with the Society of Cardiovascular Anesthesiologists: Endorsed by the Society for Cardiovascular Angiography and Interventions and the Society of Thoracic Surgeons. *Circulation*. 2006;114:e84–E231.

7. Levy WC, Mozaffarian D, Linker DT, et al. The Seattle Heart Failure Model: prediction of survival in heart failure. *Circulation*. 2006;113:1424–1433.

Chapter 3

Pathophysiology of Heart Failure

Key Points

- Heart failure is a pathophysiological state in which oxygen delivery by the heart is insufficient to meet the metabolic needs of active tissues at normal cardiac filling pressures.
- Myocardial injury or overload induces changes in ventricular structure and function that adapt to changing loading conditions in order to preserve stroke volume. This process is called *ventricular remodeling*.
- Increased myocardial wall stress and activation of neurohormonal and inflammatory systems stimulate myocellular signaling pathways for hypertrophy, fibrosis, and apoptosis, and promote ventricular remodeling and disease progression.
- The ventricular remodeling process may be favorably altered by treatment interventions that alter cardiac loading conditions and attenuate biological effects of pathological activation of neurohormonal signaling pathways.
- The clinical syndrome of heart failure is attributable to a combination of pathological changes in ventricular pump function (ventricular remodeling) coupled with alterations in peripheral oxygen utilization associated with secondary changes in vascular and skeletal muscle function.

Heart failure is a pathophysiological state that results from a mismatch between oxygen supply delivered by the heart and the metabolic demand of the body tissues. This concept of oxygen supply–demand mismatch, central to the understanding of the pathophysiology of heart failure, can be difficult to conceptualize in clinical settings. A common example of oxygen supply–demand mismatch occurs in normal physiology during vigorous exertion in normal subjects. At peak exercise in normal subjects, cardiac output reaches a maximal value (typical 4–5 times greater than resting values, or approximately 20 l/min) that limits the amounts of oxygen that can be delivered to the exercising muscles. Exhaustion of cardiac output reserve is accompanied by increasing sensations of shortness of breath and fatigue (mediated via skeletal muscle metaboreceptors), which eventually lead to cessation of exercise or reduction of exercise workload. Since the normal cardiac output reserve provides more than sufficient oxygen delivery for submaximal exertion, normal subjects rarely experience shortness of breath during routine daily activities. In patients with heart failure, reductions in cardiac output reserve and abnormalities in blood distribution and skeletal muscle oxygen metabolism lead to oxygen supply–demand mismatch at lower levels of exertion. The severity of mismatch leads to frequent symptoms of shortness of breath and fatigue during normal activities of daily living.

The majority of patients with a clinical diagnosis of heart failure have underlying changes in cardiac structure and function as the primary cause of their symptoms. However, a heart failure syndrome can occur with a completely structurally and functionally normal heart in certain settings. Severe anemia (typically, hemoglobin levels <5 gm/dl), arteriovenous shunts, and thyrotoxicosis are examples of non-cardiac conditions that can create oxygen supply–demand mismatch in the setting of a structurally and functionally normal heart. These conditions are rarely the sole cause of heart failure, but they can exacerbate heart failure symptoms in patients with underlying heart disease.

Heart failure most often occurs as a consequence of myocardial injury and/or overload (increased preload and/or afterload). The short-term response to myocardial injury is an increase in inotropic state of viable myocardium, mediated by activation of the adrenergic nervous system and the Frank Starling mechanism. The long-term response to myocardial injury and/or overload, a pathological process called ventricular remodeling, is characterized by dilation of the ventricular chamber and hypertrophy of the chamber wall.[1,2] A complex interplay of physical forces and activation of the sympathetic nervous system; the renin angiotensin aldosterone system; and other endocrine, paracrine, and autocrine signals regulate the nature of the remodeling process.[3,4] This remodeling process is fundamental to the current understanding of the pathophysiology of heart failure, as clinical measures of the severity of the remodeling process (left-ventricular ejection fraction and other measures) are strongly linked to outcomes in patients with heart failure.

The remodeling process is, in part, an adaptive response to injury or overload, since changes in cardiac structure and function preserve stroke volume and thus cardiac output reserve (Figure 3.1). The most prominent feature of remodeling in response to myocardial injury or chronic volume overload is increased left ventricle dimension (eccentric remodeling). The most prominent feature of remodeling in response to chronic pressure overload is increased left ventricle wall thickness (concentric remodeling). In many instances, a combination of eccentric and concentric remodeling is present.

The compensatory aspect of the remodeling process, preservation of stroke volume, minimizes loss of cardiac output reserve and allows most patients to remain free of signs or symptoms of heart failure. However, ventricular remodeling is inherently associated with disease progression, as ventricular dilation further increases workload (by the LaPlace relationship), and induces myocellular hypertrophy, interstitial fibrosis, and ongoing myocardial injury through apoptotic cell loss.[5] The ultimate outcome is a transition from an asymptomatic compensated state to a symptomatic decompensated state. The factors that regulate this transition are not fully characterized, but appear to be determined by the number of functioning myocytes and the length-to-width ratio of the myocytes.

Once the transition from compensated to decompensated remodeling has occurred, progressive reduction in cardiac output reserve eventually results

	Normal LV	Remodeled LV
LVEDV (ml)	100	200
LVESV (ml)	40	140
LV Stroke Volume (ml)	60	60
Ejection Fraction (%)	60	30

Figure 3.1 Effects of left-ventricular remodeling on stroke volume. Increased left-ventricular end-diastolic volume preserves left-ventricular stroke volume in the setting of reduced ejection fraction. Cardiac output reserve is theoretically normal at this stage of remodeling, but the remodeling process is inherently pathological and eventually leads to progressive hypertrophy, fibrosis, and apoptosis, with resultant loss of cardiac output reserve, and clinical heart failure.

in development of symptomatic disease. Oxygen supply–demand mismatch in exercising skeletal muscle is further exacerbated by vascular dysregulation, loss of skeletal muscle mass, and changes in skeletal muscle metabolism.[6] The net result is progressive reduction in functional capacity. Renal hypoperfusion and activation of the sympathetic nervous system, the renin angiotensin aldosterone system, and other signaling pathways promote sodium and water retention that overfills the vascular space and increases venous pressure, with consequent edema formation and other congestive signs and symptoms.[7]

An important clinical implication of this model of disease is the clear distinction between the changes in ventricular structure and function (remodeling) and the clinical syndrome of heart failure characterized by exercise intolerance and signs and symptoms of congestion. As discussed in subsequent chapters, patients with myocardial injury and/or overload often have long intervals of asymptomatic left-ventricular dysfunction that may be difficult to detect in clinical practice.

The pathophysiology of heart failure with preserved ejection fraction is largely consistent with the above discussion.[8] Certain aspects of the pathophysiology may be distinct in patients with and without hypertension (Figure 3.2). In hypertensive subjects, increased afterload induces concentric hypertrophy and reduces stroke volume, forcing the ventricle to fill on a higher portion of the diastolic pressure–volume relationship. In non-hypertensive subjects, primary changes in the diastolic pressure–volume relationship induced by progressive fibrosis or infiltrative disease force the ventricle to fill at higher pressures without a change in diastolic volumes. In both groups, reduced cardiac output reserve contributes to exercise intolerance and renal sodium and water retention with the same constellation of congestive signs and symptoms as those observed in patients with reduced ejection fraction.[9]

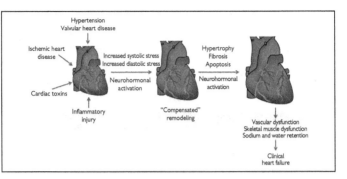

Figure 3.2 Pathophysiology of heart failure: response to myocardial injury and/or overload leads to ventricular remodeling and disease progression, and eventually clinical heart failure syndrome. This model of disease is the basis for clinical staging of disease (Chapter 4) and treatment strategies.

Treatment strategies for heart failure discussed in subsequent chapters, including the use of agents to alter loading conditions and attenuate the biological effects of pathological neurohormonal activation, are based on the presented pathophysiological model of disease.[10]

References

1. Cohn JN, Ferrari R, Sharpe N., on behalf of an international forum on cardiac remodeling. Cardiac remodeling—concepts and clinical implications: a consensus paper from an international forum on cardiac remodeling. *J Am Coll Cardiol.* 2000;35:569–582.

2. Sutton MG, Sharpe N. Left-ventricular remodeling after myocardial infarction: pathophysiology and therapy. *Circulation.* 2000;101:2981–2988.

3. Olshansky B, Sabbah HN, Hauptman PJ, Colucci WS. Parasympathetic nervous system and heart failure: pathophysiology and potential implications for therapy. *Circulation.* 2008;118:863–871.

4. Triposkiadis F, Karayannis G, Giamouzis G, Skoularigis J, Louridas G, Butler J. The sympathetic nervous system in heart failure physiology, pathophysiology, and clinical implications. *J Am Coll Cardiol.* 2009;54:1747–1762.

5. Braunwald E, Bristow MR. Congestive heart failure: fifty years of progress. *Circulation.* 2000;102:IV14–23.

6. Jackson G, Gibbs CR, Davies MK, Lip GY. ABC of heart failure. Pathophysiology. *BMJ.* 2000;320:167–170.

7. Chen HH, Schrier RW. Pathophysiology of volume overload in acute heart failure syndromes. *Am J Med.* 2006;119:S11–S16.

8. Maurer MS, King DL, El-Khoury Rumbarger L, Packer M, Burkhoff D. Left heart failure with a normal ejection fraction: identification of different pathophysiologic mechanisms. *J Card Fail.* 2005;11:177–187.

9. Katz SD, Maskin C, Jondeau G, Cocke T, Berkowitz R, LeJemtel T. Near-maximal fractional oxygen extraction by active skeletal muscle in patients with chronic heart failure. *J Appl Physiol.* 2000;88:2138–2142.

10. Koitabashi N, Kass DA. Reverse remodeling in heart failure—mechanisms and therapeutic opportunities. *Nat Rev Cardiol.* 2012;9:147–157.

Chapter 4

Clinical Staging of Heart Failure

Key Points

- The American College of Cardiology and American Heart Association staging scheme is based on the pathophysiological model of progressive ventricular remodeling in response to myocardial injury or overload.
- The New York Heart Association Classification scheme is based on the exertional symptoms reported by the patient.
- It is clinically useful to include the descriptor of ventricular function (reduced ejection fraction vs. preserved ejection fraction) in the staging of heart failure.
- It is recommended that every clinical encounter with a heart failure patient include an assessment of the stage of disease.

Determination of the stage of disease development in heart failure is clinically important, as the accurate recognition of the stage of disease provides insight into its pathophysiology and appropriate treatment. The American College of Cardiology and American Heart Association have provided a staging framework for heart failure in the consensus guidelines issued by these organizations.[1] The staging scheme was developed primarily on the basis of the current understanding of the pathophysiology of heart failure after myocardial infarction, but it can be extrapolated to heart failure with reduced ejection fraction due to other causes, or to heart failure with preserved ejection fraction. Other, more complex, staging schemes have been proposed, but none have been routinely adopted in clinical practice.[2]

The proposed staging scheme from the American College of Cardiology and American Heart Association is listed in Table 4.1. Stage A identifies patients at risk for development of heart failure. The description of the population at risk is relevant to the screening of heart failure discussed in Chapter 6, and is an acknowledgement that once structural heart disease is present, with or without symptoms, progressive remodeling will eventually lead to progressive symptoms and death. Accordingly, the best treatment for heart failure is prevention (Chapter 5). Stage B includes patients with evidence of abnormal cardiac structure and function but no limitation of functional capacity. While the left-ventricular ejection fraction is the primary measure used in most studies, the presence of left-ventricular hypertrophy also places a patient in this

Table 4.1 ACC/AHA Staging Classification

Stage	Description
Stage A: At high risk for heart failure but without structural heart disease or symptoms of heart failure.	Patients with: • hypertension • atherosclerotic disease • diabetes • obesity • metabolic syndrome • exposure to cardiotoxins • family history of cardiomyopathy
Stage B: Structural heart disease but without signs or symptoms of heart failure.	Patients with: • previous myocardial infarction • left-ventricular hypertrophy • reduced ejection fraction • asymptomatic valvular disease • other structural heart disease
Stage C: Structural heart disease with prior or current symptoms of heart failure.	Patients with: • known structural heart disease and • shortness of breath and fatigue, reduced exercise tolerance
Stage D: Refractory heart failure requiring specialized interventions.	Patients with: • marked symptoms at rest despite optimal medical therapy • recurrent hospitalizations despite optimal medical therapy

classification. Left atrial enlargement was not included in the original description of this staging scheme, but it may be the sole manifestation of structural heart disease in some patients with preserved systolic function. These patients do not have clinical symptoms of heart failure, as they are in the compensated stage of ventricular remodeling with preserved cardiac output reserve. However, these patients are at high risk for developing future symptomatic heart failure and premature death. Management of these patients is discussed in Chapter 7. Stage C includes patients with more advanced ventricular remodeling that has entered the decompensated stage with associated signs and symptoms of heart failure. Most patients present in this stage of the disease are at high risk of hospitalization and death. Management of these patients is discussed in Chapters 8 and 9. Patients who respond well to optimal therapy, with improved left-ventricular ejection fraction and/or resolution of heart failure symptoms, remain in Stage C unless there is a reasonable expectation that the initial cause of heart injury was entirely reversible (for example, acute myocarditis or peri-partum cardiomyopathy). Stage D designates patients with advanced heart failure with symptoms refractory to conventional treatment. This stage identifies a group of patients who may benefit from referral to specialized treatment centers for consideration of advanced therapies such as heart transplantation or mechanical circulatory support; or, for those patients with co-morbid conditions that preclude such advanced therapies, palliative care consultation and referral to hospice care. Management of these patients is discussed in Chapter 10.

Table 4.2 **NYHA Functional Classification. In the context assessing a patient with heart failure, the subjective assessment of functional capacity may not be closely associated with other objective assessments of the severity of cardiovascular disease, such as ejection fraction or severity of coronary artery disease. Reliable classification requires careful questioning of symptoms during specific patient activities**

Functional Capacity	Objective Assessment
Class I. Patients with cardiac disease but without resulting limitation of physical activity. Ordinary physical activity does not cause undue fatigue, palpitation, dyspnea, or anginal pain.	**A.** No objective evidence of cardiovascular disease.
Class II. Patients with cardiac disease resulting in slight limitation of physical activity. They are comfortable at rest. Ordinary physical activity results in fatigue, palpitation, dyspnea, or anginal pain.	**B.** Objective evidence of minimal cardiovascular disease.
Class III. Patients with cardiac disease resulting in marked limitation of physical activity. They are comfortable at rest. Less than ordinary activity causes fatigue, palpitation, dyspnea, or anginal pain.	**C.** Objective evidence of moderately severe cardiovascular disease.
Class IV. Patients with cardiac disease resulting in inability to carry on any physical activity without discomfort. Symptoms of heart failure or the anginal syndrome may be present even at rest. If any physical activity is undertaken, discomfort is increased.	**D.** Objective evidence of severe cardiovascular disease.

Characterization of the functional capacity of the patient should be assessed at every clinical encounter as an integral part of the staging process. The most commonly used staging scheme for functional capacity is the New York Heart Association criteria (Table 4.2).[3] These categories are very broad and require careful questioning of the patient for accurate assignment. Specific questions on their ability to perform daily activities such as bathing, dressing, household or yard chores, leisure activities (golf, bowling, tennis, etc.), walking up stairs, and walking on flat ground are useful to characterize functional capacity. A questionnaire for determination of New York Heart Association Class has been validated for use in research settings, but it has not been widely adopted in clinical settings.[4] Other measures of functional capacity (Canadian Cardiovascular Society Functional Classification and Specific Activity Scale) have not been widely adopted in heart failure populations.[5]

Finally, it is clinically useful to include the descriptor of ventricular function (reduced ejection fraction vs. preserved ejection fraction) in the staging of heart failure, as treatment strategies depend on the ventricular function.

Every clinical encounter with a heart failure patient should include a summary statement on staging in the assessment section of the medical record in accordance with the following suggested format:

"Patient has heart failure associated with (reduced/preserved) ejection fraction, AHA/ACC Stage (A/B/C/D), NYHA Class (I,II,III,IV)."

References

1. Hunt SA, Abraham WT, Chin MH, et al. ACC/AHA 2005 Guideline Update for the Diagnosis and Management of Chronic Heart Failure in the Adult: A Report of the American College of Cardiology/American Heart Association Task Force on Practice Guidelines (writing committee to update the 2001 guidelines for the evaluation and management of heart failure): Developed in collaboration with the American College of Chest Physicians and the International Society for Heart and Lung Transplantation: Endorsed by the Heart Rhythm Society. *Circulation.* 2005;112:e154–e235.

2. Field ML, Coats AJ. Grading, staging and scoring of left-ventricular hypertrophy, left-ventricular dilatation, asymptomatic left-ventricular dysfunction and chronic heart failure. *Eur Heart J.* 1999;20:1224–1233.

3. Criteria Committee of the New York Heart Association. *Nomenclature and Criteria for Diagnosis of Diseases of the Heart and Great Vessels.* Boston, MA: Little, Brown & Co.; 1994.

4. Kubo SH, Schulman S, Starling RC, Jessup M, Wentworth D, Burkhoff D. Development and validation of a patient questionnaire to determine New York Heart Association classification. *J Card Fail.* 2004;10:228–235.

5. Goldman L, Hashimoto B, Cook EF, Loscalzo A. Comparative reproducibility and validity of systems for assessing cardiovascular functional class: advantages of a new specific activity scale. *Circulation.* 1981;64:1227–1234.

Chapter 5

Prevention of Heart Failure

Key Points

- An estimated 65 million patients are at risk for developing heart failure in the United States.
- Primary prevention therapies aimed at reducing risk of myocardial infarction are recommended to reduce risk of heart failure.
- Effective treatment of hypertension reduces the risk of heart failure development.

Stage A of the AHA/ACC heart failure staging classification identifies asymptomatic patients without structural heart disease at increased risk for future development of heart failure. It is estimated that 65 million Americans are in this group, and that 550,000 new cases of heart failure are identified each year. These asymptomatic patients are generally treated in primary care practices, or they may not be seeking medical care. Effective preventive treatment in this group should be a high priority, since once structural heart disease is evident, available treatments slow disease progression and improve outcomes, but do not provide a curative remedy. Accordingly, the importance of prevention efforts in primary care settings cannot be overemphasized.[1]

There are multiple barriers to effective hypertensive treatment attributable to patient factors, physician factors, and systems factors. *Clinical inertia*, defined as "failure to adjust hypertensive therapy at clinical encounters with recorded blood pressure above consensus guideline goal," has been identified as a frequent problem in the management of hypertension patients.[2] Although the factors that contribute to clinical inertia are complex, one important component is the asymptomatic nature of hypertension, with consequent patient resistance to the initiation or intensification of therapy. The clinician must educate and motivate the patient to adhere to recommended treatments. Established symptomatic heart failure carries a one- and five-year prognosis worse than that of many cancers. If an appropriate analogy between cancer prevention and heart failure prevention were made evident to patients, patient resistance to appropriate hypertension treatment might be reduced.

For most patients, preventive strategies are directed towards reducing the risk of myocardial injury (primary prevention of myocardial infarction) and maintaining normal loading conditions on the heart (hypertension management).[1]

Primary prevention of myocardial infarction is an important strategy for preventing heart failure. The therapeutic strategy should include appropriate

lifestyle modifications (diet, weight loss, exercise) and pharmacological management. Clinical trials of 3-hydroxy-3-methyl-glutaryl-CoA reductase (HMG-CoA)
reductase inhibitors have demonstrated significant reduction of heart failure risk
when compared with placebo.[3] Strategies for management of hyperlipidemia
should be conducted in accord with consensus guidelines.[4] The role of aspirin
for primary prevention of myocardial infarction remains controversial and may
be considered on an individual basis in higher risk patients.[5,6] In patients with
established coronary heart disease, revascularization may be considered on an
individual basis, but the evidence that revascularization prevents subsequent
heart failure development is not conclusive.[7]

Treatment of hypertension is important for the prevention of heart failure
beyond its effects on reducing the risk of myocardial infarction (Figure 5.1).
Clinical trials that utilized primarily beta-adrenergic receptor blockers and thiazide diuretics demonstrated large reductions in new onset of heart failure when
compared with placebo.[3] Subsequent clinical trials have demonstrated that
the risk of heart failure during treatment is comparable among most available
classes of anti-hypertensive agents. In the Antihypertensive and Lipid-Lowering
Treatment to Prevent Heart Attack Trial (ALLHAT), the alpha-blocking agent
doxazosin arm of the study was stopped prematurely, due to increased incidence of heart failure in this group when compared with the other randomized treatment arms.[8] Although interpretation of this finding is limited by the
adjudication process used in this trial and the absence of a placebo control
group, alpha blockers should not be used as first-line anti-hypertensive therapy in patients felt to be at high risk for development of heart failure. The
angiotensin-converting enzyme inhibitor ramipril reduced risk of heart failure
by 23% compared with placebo in patients at high risk for heart failure but no
known left-ventricular systolic dysfunction.[9] Approximately half of the patients
in this study had a history of prior myocardial infarction. The choice of anti-
hypertensive agent and blood pressure goals of therapy should be individualized
according to patient comorbidities per consensus guidelines.[10]

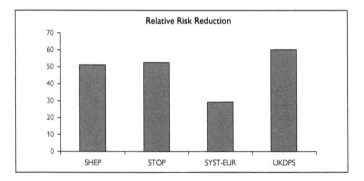

Figure 5.1 Effect of hypertension therapy vs. placebo on risk of heart failure (adapted
from reference 3). Anti-hypertensive regimens varied among trials, but a significant
reduction in risk of heart failure was observed in all trials. Effective treatment of hypertension is one of the most important interventions for prevention of heart failure.

Treatment of other risk factors for myocardial infarction (smoking, obesity, diabetes mellitus) has not been shown to reduce heart failure incidence in clinical trials. The effect of tighter glycemic control on risk of heart failure was neutral in the United Kingdom Prospective Diabetes Study (UKPDS) trial and increased in the Action to Control Cardiovascular Risk in Diabetes (ACCORD) trial.[11,12] The safety of thiazolidinediones and metformin in heart failure patients with diabetes remains uncertain.[13,14] There are no randomized trials to determine the effects of smoking cessation and weight loss on risk of heart failure, but these interventions are recommended.

Patients exposed to cardiotoxic agents during cancer chemotherapy are at greater lifelong risk of developing heart failure. Reduced use of anthracyclines (or switching to the use of recently developed liposomal forms of anthracyclines), increased use of cardioprotective agents, and the development of more sensitive surveillance techniques, including imaging and biomarkers, may reduce the risk of heart failure in this population.[15]

For patients with known moderate to severe valvular heart disease, existing guidelines describe diagnostic and treatment strategies for the prevention of heart failure. These patients should be followed in conjunction with a cardiologist.[16]

References

1. Schocken DD, Benjamin EJ, Fonarow GC, et al. Prevention of heart failure: A scientific statement from the American Heart Association Councils on Epidemiology and Prevention, Clinical Cardiology, Cardiovascular Nursing, and High Blood Pressure Research; Quality of Care and Outcomes Research Interdisciplinary Working Group; and Functional Genomics and Translational Biology Interdisciplinary Working Group. *Circulation*. 2008;117:2544–2565.

2. Faria C, Wenzel M, Lee KW, Coderre K, Nichols J, Belletti DA. A narrative review of clinical inertia: focus on hypertension. *JASH*. 2009;3:267–276.

3. Baker DW. Prevention of heart failure. *J Card Fail*. 2002;8:333–346.

4. Third report of the National Cholesterol Education Program (NCEP) expert panel on detection, evaluation, and treatment of high blood cholesterol in adults (Adult Treatment Panel III) final report. *Circulation*. 2002;106:3143–3421.

5. Berger JS, Lala A, Krantz MJ, Baker GS, Hiatt WR. Aspirin for the prevention of cardiovascular events in patients without clinical cardiovascular disease: a meta-analysis of randomized trials. *Am Heart J*. July, 2011;162(1):115–124.e2.

6. Collaborative meta-analysis of randomised trials of antiplatelet therapy for prevention of death, myocardial infarction, and stroke in high risk patients. *BMJ*. 2002;324:71–86.

7. Bonow RO, Maurer G, Lee KL, et al. Myocardial viability and survival in ischemic left ventricular dysfunction. *N Engl J Med*. 2011;364:1617–1625.

8. Major outcomes in high-risk hypertensive patients randomized to angiotensin-converting enzyme inhibitor or calcium channel blocker vs. diuretic: The Antihypertensive and Lipid-Lowering Treatment to Prevent Heart Attack Trial (ALLHAT). *JAMA*. 2002;288:2981–2997.

9. Yusuf S, Sleight P, Pogue J, Bosch J, Davies R, Dagenais G. Effects of an angiotensin-converting-enzyme inhibitor, ramipril, on cardiovascular events in high-risk patients. The Heart Outcomes Prevention Evaluation Study investigators. *N Engl J Med*. 2000;342:145–153.

10. Chobanian AV, Bakris GL, Black HR, et al. Seventh report of the Joint National Committee on Prevention, Detection, Evaluation, and Treatment of High Blood Pressure. *Hypertension*. 2003;42:1206–1252.

11. Intensive blood-glucose control with sulphonylureas or insulin compared with conventional treatment and risk of complications in patients with type 2 diabetes (UKPDS 33). UK Prospective Diabetes Study (UKPDS) group. *Lancet*. 1998;352:837–853.

12. Gerstein HC, Miller ME, Byington RP, et al. Effects of intensive glucose lowering in type 2 diabetes. *N Engl J Med*. 2008;358:2545–2559.

13. Hernandez AV, Usmani A, Rajamanickam A, Moheet A. Thiazolidinediones and risk of heart failure in patients with or at high risk of type 2 diabetes mellitus: a meta-analysis and meta-regression analysis of placebo-controlled randomized clinical trials. *Am J Cardiovasc Drugs*. 2011;11:115–128.

14. Aguilar D, Chan W, Bozkurt B, Ramasubbu K, Deswal A. Metformin use and mortality in ambulatory patients with diabetes and heart failure. *Circulation: Heart Failure*. 2011;4:53–58.

15. Gianni L, Herman EH, Lipshultz SE, Minotti G, Sarvazyan N, Sawyer DB. Anthracycline cardiotoxicity: from bench to bedside. *J Clin Oncol*. 2008;26:3777–3784.

16. Bonow RO, Carabello BA, Kanu C, et al. ACC/AHA 2006 guidelines for the management of patients with valvular heart disease: a report of the American College of Cardiology/American Heart Association task force on practice guidelines (writing committee to revise the 1998 guidelines for the management of patients with valvular heart disease): developed in collaboration with the Society of Cardiovascular Anesthesiologists: endorsed by the Society for Cardiovascular Angiography and Interventions and the Society of Thoracic Surgeons. *Circulation*. 2006;114:e84–e231.

Chapter 6

Screening for Heart Failure

Key Points

- There are no proven cost-effective imaging or laboratory testing strategies for screening for asymptomatic left-ventricular dysfunction in primary care populations.
- Echocardiography is the most common screening modality used for detection of left-ventricular dysfunction, and can be applied in selected patients with abnormal signs and symptoms suggestive of heart failure, patients with new abnormalities on electrocardiograms, and patients with cardiomegaly on chest radiography.
- In selected patients with risk factors for left-ventricular dysfunction, brain natriuretic peptide testing can be useful to exclude left-ventricular dysfunction.

There are an estimated 65 million patients in AHA/ACC Stage A (patients at increased risk for heart failure), and approximately 550,000 new cases of heart failure in the United States each year (combined Stages B, C, and D). Presumably, the bulk of the incident cases of heart failure are in Stage C, as clinical detection typically occurs after the onset of symptoms. Given the pathophysiological model for heart failure presented in Chapter 3, it is likely that many more undetected asymptomatic patients are present in the population of patients at risk.[1] Due to the relatively low incidence of left-ventricular dysfunction in the at-risk population (conservatively, less than 10%, including symptomatic and asymptomatic cases), screening tests with extremely high accuracy would be required to be clinically useful (per Bayes's Theorem). Alternatively, clinical skills can be used to identify subgroups of patients at increased risk, with judicious use of additional testing in selected patients.

There are no proven strategies for routine screening for asymptomatic left-ventricular dysfunction (Stage B patients) in the general population. By definition, these patients have abnormal left-ventricular structure but no symptoms of heart failure.

Echocardiography is the most commonly used imaging modality for detection of abnormal left-ventricular structure and/or function. In a random sample of community dwelling individuals in Olmstead County, Minnesota, echocardiographic screening demonstrated that 34% of the population with no symptoms of heart failure had echocardiographic evidence of some degree of left-ventricular dysfunction consistent with Stage B heart failure.[2] The prevalence of abnormal left-ventricular function and clinical heart failure was increased with increasing age (Figure 6.1). However, the majority of cardiac abnormalities identified in this study sample were related to echocardiographic indices of abnormal diastolic function; reduced left-ventricular ejection fraction (defined as less than 50%) or left-ventricular hypertrophy was detected in under 10% of the population. The clinical utility of identification of diastolic dysfunction by echocardiographic criteria is uncertain, as the clinical outcomes of the Stage B patients identified in this study did not differ from those of a control population with no risk factors for heart disease. The relatively high proportion of clinically silent reduced ejection fraction detected in this cross-sectional study may also be attributed to the cumulative effects of a low annual incidence, and is consistent with observations of a long period of asymptomatic left-ventricular dysfunction after myocardial infarction (Chapter 2). The cross-sectional design of the study limits the ability to determine the clinical utility of echocardiographic screening during longitudinal ambulatory care settings. In clinical practice, assessment of left-ventricular function is a guideline recommended procedure after myocardial infarction, so the group with post-myocardial left-ventricular dysfunction comprises the majority of Stage B patients. Other scenarios where echocardiography screening may be reasonable include evaluation of certain new EKG abnormalities (evidence of new Q-wave myocardial infarction, left bundle branch block, and/or left-ventricular hypertrophy) in asymptomatic patients, evaluation of an enlarged cardiac silhouette on chest imaging, or as part of the evaluation for non–heart failure cardiac symptoms such as palpitations, syncope, or chest pain. Despite the increased prevalence of asymptomatic structural heart disease in the elderly, there is no current evidence to support routine echocardiography screening procedures in this population.

Brain natriuretic peptide (BNP) is a cardiac-derived peptide hormone that is secreted by myocytes (primarily in the left ventricle) in response to increased wall tension.[3] BNP is produced in the heart as a longer pro-hormone peptide chain, and then processed for secretion as both the active 32 amino acid hormone and inactive N-terminal peptide (NT-proBNP). The biological

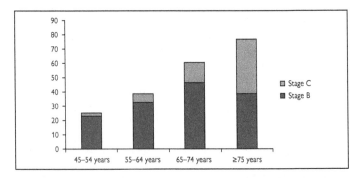

Figure 6.1 Prevalence of Stage B and Stage C heart failure by age in residents of Olmstead County, Minn. (Adapted from Mosterd A, Hoes AW, de Bruyne MC, et al., Prevalence of heart failure and left-ventricular dysfunction in the general population; the Rotterdam Study. *Eur Heart J*, 1999;20:447–455.)

actions of BNP (vasodilation, increased renal sodium excretion) are mediated by membrane-bound natriuretic peptide receptors in target tissues. In heart failure patients, BNP is considered a counter-regulatory hormone, secreted by the heart in response to volume overload induced by the activation of the renin-angiotensin-aldosterone system, sympathetic nervous system, and vasopressin. Increased levels of BNP (and NT-proBNP) are associated with greater impairment of functional capacity and greater mortality risk in patients with symptomatic heart failure. In a random sample of ambulatory patients from primary care practices in Scotland, left-ventricular systolic dysfunction (defined as left-ventricular ejection fraction <30% as measured by echocardiography) was identified in 3% of the population.[4] BNP levels were higher in these patients (with or without symptoms of heart failure), but the positive predictive value of the test was low, even in the higher-risk group with a history of ischemic heart disease. A smaller population-based study in elderly subjects from the United Kingdom demonstrated that BNP measurements were most useful for their high negative predictive value (ruling out left-ventricular systolic dysfunction), with low positive predictive value.[5] These two investigations were limited to the detection of left-ventricular systolic dysfunction. In the Framingham study population, measurement of plasma BNP was not useful as a screening test for detecting abnormal left-ventricular structure (reduced ejection fraction or left-ventricular hypertrophy), even in subgroups with clinical markers of increased risk.[6] Other biomarkers of left-ventricular dysfunction and heart failure are in development or clinically available (galectin-3), but their clinical utility for screening for asymptomatic left-ventricular systolic dysfunction has not been determined.[7]

Based on available data, there are no imaging or laboratory tests that can be recommended for routine screening for detection of abnormal left-ventricular structure or function in asymptomatic patients. Careful history and physical examination are important tools in clinical practice, with special attention given to patients with multiple risk factors for heart failure, and patients with abnormal cardiac exam, or any unexplained signs of congestion. Given the known

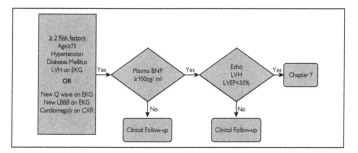

Figure 6.2 Proposed algorithm for screening asymptomatic left-ventricular dysfunction. This algorithm is based on extrapolations from existing epidemiological and clinical trial data but has not been prospectively tested in clinical trials. The clinical utility of the algorithm with respect to impact on clinical outcomes is unknown. However, clinical trials have identified therapies can benefit selected patients with asymptomatic left-ventricular dysfunction (see Chapter 7).

increased risk of adverse outcomes in patients with abnormal left-ventricular structure or function, and the availability of specific therapies known to reduce this risk of adverse outcomes (discussed in Chapter 7), judicious use of echocardiography is reasonable in selected patients. A suggested algorithm for use of echocardiography in asymptomatic patients is provided in Figure 6.2.

References

1. Mosterd A, Hoes AW, de Bruyne MC, et al. Prevalence of heart failure and left-ventricular dysfunction in the general population; the Rotterdam Study. *Eur Heart J*. 1999;20:447–455.

2. Ammar KA, Jacobsen SJ, Mahoney DW, et al. Prevalence and prognostic significance of heart failure stages: application of the American College of Cardiology/American Heart Association heart failure staging criteria in the community. *Circulation*. 2007;115:1563–1570.

3. de Lemos JA, McGuire DK, Drazner MH. B-type natriuretic peptide in cardiovascular disease. *Lancet*. 2003;362:316–322.

4. McDonagh TA, Robb SD, Murdoch DR, et al. Biochemical detection of left-ventricular systolic dysfunction. *Lancet*. 1998;351:9–13.

5. Smith H, Pickering RM, Struthers A, Simpson I, Mant D. Biochemical diagnosis of ventricular dysfunction in elderly patients in general practice: Observational study. *BMJ*. 2000;320:906–908.

6. Vasan RS, Benjamin EJ, Larson MG, et al. Plasma natriuretic peptides for community screening for left-ventricular hypertrophy and systolic dysfunction: the Framingham Heart Study. *JAMA*. 2002;288:1252–1259.

7. Braunwald E. Biomarkers in heart failure. *N Engl J Med*. 2008;358:2148–2159.

Chapter 7

Management of Asymptomatic Left-Ventricular Dysfunction

Key Points

- Asymptomatic patients with evidence of left-ventricular systolic dysfunction (left-ventricular ejection fraction <50% and/or left-ventricular hypertrophy) are at increased risk for cardiovascular morbidity and mortality.
- Asymptomatic left-ventricular systolic dysfunction (left-ventricular ejection fraction <50%) is most often identified after an index myocardial infarction.
- Asymptomatic left-ventricular hypertrophy (determined by echocardiography or cardiac magnetic resonance imaging) is most often identified in patients with a history of hypertension and/or chronic kidney disease.
- A report of "diastolic dysfunction" on an echocardiogram or modestly elevated brain natriuretic peptide is not sufficient to make a diagnosis of asymptomatic heart failure with preserved ejection fraction.
- A combined neurohormonal antagonist regimen (angiotensin-converting enzyme inhibitor and beta-adrenergic receptor blocker) is reasonable to consider for asymptomatic patients with reduced ejection fraction.
- A multi-drug regimen including inhibitors of the renin-angiotensin aldosterone system is reasonable to control blood pressure in asymptomatic left-ventricular hypertrophy in patients with preserved ejection fraction.

Clinical Diagnosis

Once left-ventricular dysfunction has been identified by an imaging procedure (most commonly, transthoracic echocardiography), the patient should be carefully questioned about their daily activities and symptoms of heart failure. Patients with "asymptomatic" left-ventricular systolic dysfunction are known to have reduced peak aerobic capacity when compared with age-matched controls.[1] The state of being "asymptomatic" is highly dependent on the level of exertion in daily activities. Many patients interpret deterioration in exercise capability as a normal part of aging, or due to obesity or deconditioning, and may not offer complaints unless directly questioned. Patients also tend to spontaneously curtail physical activities that produce symptoms of dyspnea, and continue to consider themselves "asymptomatic" in spite of these self-imposed activity restrictions. It is useful to ask close-ended questions about specific activities to obtain a detailed description of the level of aerobic stress in patient activities of daily living. To identify truly asymptomatic patients (and accurately distinguish Class B vs. Class C patients), the questions should focus on more strenuous activities at home (gardening, home improvement, cleaning chores, sports) and work (if relevant to the patient's occupation) and on any recent change in their perceived ability to perform activities, or any shift to a more sedentary lifestyle. A detailed history for risk factors for heart disease, presence of systemic inflammatory disease or other chronic diseases, and exposure to known cardiotoxins (excessive alcohol intake or cancer chemotherapy) should also be obtained.

Confirmatory Testing

Asymptomatic left-ventricular systolic dysfunction (left-ventricular ejection fraction <50%) is most often identified after an index myocardial infarction. In these patients, the etiology of left-ventricular systolic dysfunction is attributable to the underlying coronary artery disease. In patients with chance discovery of unsuspected left-ventricular systolic dysfunction, a clinical evaluation to identify the possible cause of left-ventricular dysfunction should be undertaken in accord with the discussion in Chapter 8.

Asymptomatic left-ventricular hypertrophy (determined by echocardiography or cardiac magnetic resonance imaging [MRI]) is most often identified in patients with a history of hypertension and/or chronic kidney disease. In the Framingham population, increased left-ventricular mass was detected by echocardiography in 16% of asymptomatic men (mean age 55 years) and 21% of asymptomatic women (mean age 57 years).[2] Transthoracic echocardiography reports may describe "diastolic dysfunction" based on the temporal pattern of mitral valve diastolic flow detected by Doppler echocardiography and tissue Doppler measurements of the velocity of movement of the mitral annulus. A finding of a pseudonormalized or restrictive pattern of mitral valve inflow is not by itself sufficient to make a diagnosis symptomatic or asymptomatic heart failure, but it should prompt a careful assessment for evidence of congestive signs and symptoms. The presence of left-atrial enlargement in association with abnormal mitral valve inflow increases the likelihood that the patient may have an early form of heart failure, but in the absence of changes in left-ventricular structure and function, this does not meet criteria for American College of Cardiology/American Heart Association Stage B. Regardless of the formal staging, these changes on echocardiogram are likely to indicate an increased risk of heart failure and merit a careful evaluation for signs and symptoms of congestion, and treatment of risk factors as described below.

In addition to studies directed at determining the etiology of left-ventricular dysfunction, all patients should undergo a detailed physical examination to document any signs of congestion and/or cardiac enlargement, 12-lead electrocardiogram, chest X-ray, comprehensive metabolic panel, iron studies, thyroid function tests, and complete blood count. There is no proven role for routine assessment of brain natriuretic peptide in asymptomatic patients. However, measurement of brain natriuretic peptide could be considered in patients with comorbid condition(s) that limit exercise capacity (peripheral vascular, pulmonary, neuromuscular, or joint diseases) in order to assess whether the patient is "asymptomatic" from the cardiac standpoint. Brain natriuretic peptide is most useful for its negative predictive value; a value in the normal range makes a diagnosis of heart failure unlikely (except in obese subjects). Moderate elevations of natriuretic peptide above the normal range are non-specific and are not sufficient to make a diagnosis of heart failure in the absence of clinical signs or symptoms of congestion.

Some patients may have limited exercise tolerance primarily related to non-cardiac comorbidities such as obesity, deconditioning, lung disease, neurological disease, or joint disease. Pulmonary function tests and cardiopulmonary exercise testing can be used to differentiate cardiac vs. non-cardiac limitations to exercise.

If the diagnosis remains in doubt despite careful clinical assessment and non-invasive testing, right-heart catheterization may be considered to measure cardiac filling pressures in a patient with preserved ejection fraction and exercise intolerance of uncertain cause (unable to perform a stress test due to comorbidities, or equivocal stress test results).[3] Simultaneous measurements of right- and left-ventricular pressures should be considered in patients with other clinical features suggestive of restrictive cardiomyopathy. Cardiac filling pressures should be measured at rest and during exercise if possible, or at a minimum in response to an acute volume load (lifting the lower extremities, or saline infusion). Abnormal elevation of cardiac filling pressures at rest and/ or during exercise strongly suggests that cardiac dysfunction is contributing to exercise intolerance.

Risk Stratification

Risk of cardiovascular morbidity and mortality is increased in patients with evidence of structural heart disease (reduced ejection fraction and/or left-ventricular hypertrophy).[2,4,5] Risk is directly proportional to the severity of the structural abnormality in the heart. Once abnormal left-ventricular structure has been identified in an asymptomatic patient, it is reasonable to reassess cardiac structure and function if symptoms appear, or otherwise at two-year intervals.

The appearance of symptoms of exercise intolerance (transition from Stage B to Stage C) is an important marker of disease progression and increased risk for adverse clinical outcomes. Patients should be carefully questioned at each visit to determine if there is any evidence of a worsening of exercise capacity. If there is uncertainty about a change in symptoms, exercise testing can provide an objective assessment of aerobic capacity.

Biomarkers such as brain natriuretic peptide may provide additional prognostic information, but are not recommended for routine screening of asymptomatic patients. This biomarker can be used if there is uncertainty about any change in symptoms, or to further evaluate new onset of dyspnea in patients with comorbid conditions that limit exercise capacity as described above.

Treatment Strategies

Lifestyle modifications, including moderate aerobic exercise, weight reduction, reduction of dietary fat and sodium, and smoking cessation, should be recommended to all asymptomatic patients with left-ventricular dysfunction.

Asymptomatic patients with left-ventricular systolic dysfunction have evidence of neurohormonal activation when compared with age-matched control subjects.[6] Clinical trial data support the use of neurohormonal antagonists in this population as described below.

All asymptomatic patients with reduced ejection fraction should be treated with an angiotensin-converting enzyme inhibitor if possible. A summary of the clinical trials in support of this recommendation is provided in Table 7.1.[7–9] Overall, these trials provide concordant evidence of the clinical benefit of angiotensin-converting enzyme inhibition in asymptomatic patients with reduced left-ventricular ejection fraction. The greatest proportion of the data for asymptomatic subjects is derived from the Studies of Left Ventricular Dysfunction (SOLVD) prevention trial, as this trial only enrolled patients without heart failure symptoms, whereas 40% to 60% of the patients in the Survival and Ventricular Enlargement (SAVE) and Trandolapril Cardiac Evaluation (TRACE) studies had at least transient heart failure in the post-myocardial infarction setting. Although the 8% reduction in total mortality in the SOLVD prevention trial was not statistically significant, enalapril therapy did significantly reduce the combined risk of death and new onset of heart failure by 29% and did significantly reduce the risk of heart failure hospitalization by 20%, compared with placebo. Moreover, evaluation of longer-term survival after a mean follow-up of 11 years demonstrated a significant 14% reduction in all-cause mortality in patients treated with enalapril when compared with placebo.[10] There are few available data on the effects of angiotensin-converting enzyme inhibition in asymptomatic patients with reduced ejection fraction due to non-ischemic causes. In the SOLVD prevention study, the benefits of enalapril vs. placebo did not differ among the 20% of patients without history of myocardial infarction compared with the 80% of patients with history of myocardial infarction.[7] For all the studies referenced in Table 7.1, therapy was initiated at least three days after acute myocardial infarction at a low dose and gradually titrated over weeks or months as tolerated to the target dose. Earlier initiation of angiotensin-converting enzyme inhibition therapy after myocardial infarction is not recommended due to increased risk of adverse events.[11] Since the endpoint of therapy is reduction in mortality risk, it is recommended to attempt titration to the target dose listed in Table 7.1 as tolerated. Approximately 60% to 80% of the patients in these studies did receive the target dose of therapy. Other angiotensin-converting enzyme inhibitors not listed in Table 7.1 may also be considered for use in this population at doses demonstrated to be associated with reduction in adverse outcomes in post-myocardial infarction or chronic left-ventricular systolic dysfunction trials.[12,13] A meta-analysis of the angiotensin-converting enzyme inhibitors studies in post-myocardial infarction populations demonstrated an absolute risk reduction of mortality of 2.3% compared with placebo, yielding a number needed to treat for one year to save one life of

Table 7.1 Summary of placebo-controlled, double-blind, randomized clinical trials of angiotensin-converting enzyme inhibitors in patients with asymptomatic left-ventricular systolic dysfunction

Study Acronym	N	Active Drug	Mean LVEF	Mean Follow-up (months)	Start Dose	Target Dose	Morta-lity RR
SOLVD-Prevention[6]	4228	Enalapril	28%	37	2.5 mg BID	10 mg BID	8%
SAVE[8]	2231	Captopril	31	42	6.25 mg TID	50 mg TID	19%
TRACE[7]	1749	Trandolapril	<35%	24–50	1 mg daily	4 mg daily	22%

43 patients.[13] The most common side effects of angiotensin-converting enzyme inhibition in all trials were symptomatic hypotension, worsening renal function, hyperkalemia, and cough. Risk of some side effects can be minimized by selecting patients with systolic blood pressure >110 mmHg, estimated creatinine clearance >60 ml/min, and serum potassium <5.0 meq/l. Serum creatinine and serum potassium should be monitored at initiation of therapy, up-titration of therapy, and periodically during chronic therapy. For patients with cough in response angiotensin-converting enzyme inhibition therapy, the angiotensin receptor antagonist valsartan (initial dose 20 mg twice daily, target dose 80 mg twice daily) was shown to be as effective as captopril for reduction in mortality risk in asymptomatic and symptomatic patients with reduced left-ventricular dysfunction after myocardial infarction.[14]

Asymptomatic patients with post-myocardial infarction left-ventricular systolic dysfunction should also be treated with a beta-adrenergic receptor blocker. Most of the clinical trials of beta-blockers in acute myocardial infarction were conducted before the development of modern reperfusion therapies, anti-platelet therapies, and angiotensin-converting enzyme inhibition therapy. In the Carvedilol Post-Infarct Survival Control in Left Ventricular Dysfunction (CAPRICORN) study, the beta-adrenergic receptor blocking agent carvedilol (initial dose 6.25 mg twice daily, target dose 25 mg twice daily) was compared to placebo in 1,959 post-myocardial infarction patients with left-ventricular ejection fraction <40% who received standard therapies including angiotensin-converting enzyme inhibition and anti-platelet therapies in >85% and thrombolysis or primary angioplasty in 45%.[15] The mean left-ventricular ejection fraction was 32%. Subjects with and without heart failure symptoms were enrolled; approximately 30% were treated with intravenous diuretics at the time of randomization. Carvedilol therapy was associated with a 23% reduction in all-cause mortality (a 2.3% absolute risk reduction, corresponding to a number needed to treat for one year to save one life of 43 patients). In this study, carvedilol therapy was started a minimum of three days after the index myocardial infarction and was titrated slowly to the target dose at three- to 10-day intervals. Carvedilol was well tolerated with this regimen, and 74% of the subjects reached the target dose of 25 mg twice daily. In contrast to other post-myocardial infarction beta-adrenergic receptor blocker trials,[16] there was no observed excess risk of heart failure associated with carvedilol therapy compared with placebo; in fact, an opposite trend towards reduction of heart failure risk compared with placebo was observed in this study. To minimize the risk of adverse side effects in clinical practice, beta-adrenergic receptor blockers should be initiated during periods of clinical stability, with slow upward titration as tolerated. Since the clinical endpoint for beta-adrenergic receptor blocker therapy is reduction of mortality risk, an attempt should be made to titrate to the maximum tolerated dose. Although other beta-blockers have been shown to reduce mortality post-myocardial infarction (propranolol and timolol), none have been tested in clinical trials of patients who have received reperfusion therapy. Accordingly, it is reasonable to preferentially use carvedilol in patients with asymptomatic left-ventricular systolic dysfunction due to past myocardial infarction. There are no available data in asymptomatic patients with left-ventricular systolic dysfunction due to non-ischemic causes, but it is reasonable to use carvedilol at the same dosing regimen in this population.

Asymptomatic patients with left-ventricular hypertrophy associated with chronic hypertension will often require multiple drugs for the control of blood pressure. Regression of left-ventricular hypertrophy with anti-hypertensive treatment is achievable and is associated with a reduced risk of adverse outcomes. In a meta-analysis of hypertension treatment trials with serial echocardiographic measurement of left-ventricular mass (Figure 7.1), angiotensin-receptor blockers, angiotensin-converting enzyme inhibitors, and calcium channel blockers were associated with greater reduction of left-ventricular mass (9%–12%) when compared with beta-adrenergic receptor blockers (5%).[17] Diuretics had an intermediate effect on reduction of left-ventricular mass (6%).

Two important large randomized clinical trials were excluded from this meta-analysis. The Treatment of Mild Hypertension Study (TOMHS) demonstrated that diuretic therapy with chlorthalidone as monotherapy was associated with the greatest reduction in left-ventricular mass (34%), compared with other hypertension drug classes as monotherapy (including beta-adrenergic receptor blocker [23%], calcium channel blocker [25%], alpha-adrenergic receptor blocker [24%] and angiotensin-converting enzyme inhibitor [23%]).[18] Importantly, the placebo group in this study, in which lifestyle change (weight loss, increased exercise, dietary sodium reduction, and decreased alcohol intake) was the only intervention, achieved a 27% reduction in left-ventricular mass, an effect not different from the active treatment groups, despite smaller reduction in blood pressure. The Losartan Intervention For Endpoint reduction (LIFE) study randomly assigned 9193 subjects with hypertension and electrocardiographic evidence of left-ventricular hypertrophy to treatment with either losartan (50 mg–100 mg with addition of hydrochlorothiazide as needed) or atenolol (50 mg–100 mg with addition of hydrochlorothiazide as needed).[19] Despite comparable reductions in blood pressure, losartan therapy was associated with a significant reduction in the risk of the combined endpoint of cardiovascular death, non-fatal stroke, and non-fatal myocardial infarction. Losartan therapy was also associated with a greater reduction of electrocardiographic evidence of left-ventricular hypertrophy, compared with atenolol. Application of the findings from the meta-analysis and these two additional clinical trials to clinical practice is limited by the emphasis on monotherapy in clinical trials, as distinct from the use of multiple classes of drugs in clinical practice.

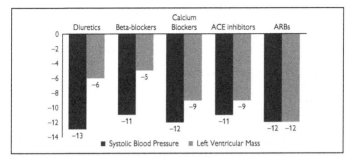

Figure 7.1 Percent reduction in systolic blood pressure and left-ventricular mass in response to different classes of anti-hypertensive therapy (adapted from reference 15). Despite comparable reductions in blood pressure, beta-adrenergic receptor blocker therapy was associated with less regression of left-ventricular mass, compared with calcium blockers, ACE inhibitors, and ARBs.

Taken together, it is reasonable to preferentially use classes of anti-hypertensive agents other than beta-adrenergic receptor blockers in patients with evidence of left-ventricular hypertrophy and no other compelling indication for beta-adrenergic receptor blocker therapy. It is also important to emphasize the benefits of lifestyle modification in this patient population.

References

1. LeJemtel TH, Liang CS, Stewart DK, et al. Reduced peak aerobic capacity in asymptomatic left-ventricular systolic dysfunction. A substudy of the Studies of Left-Ventricular Dysfunction (SOLVD). SOLVD investigator. *Circulation*. 1994;90:2757–2760.

2. Levy D, Garrison RJ, Savage DD, Kannel WB, Castelli WP. Prognostic implications of echocardiographically determined left-ventricular mass in the Framingham heart study. *N Engl J Med*. 1990;322:1561–1566.

3. Borlaug BA, Nishimura RA, Sorajja P, Lam CS, Redfield MM. Exercise hemodynamics enhance diagnosis of early heart failure with preserved ejection fraction. *Circ. Heart Fail*. 2010;3:588–595.

4. Lauer MS, Evans JC, Levy D. Prognostic implications of subclinical left-ventricular dilatation and systolic dysfunction in men free of overt cardiovascular disease (the Framingham heart study). *Am J Cardiol*. 1992;70:1180–1184.

5. Levy D, Salomon M, D'Agostino RB, Belanger AJ, Kannel WB. Prognostic implications of baseline electrocardiographic features and their serial changes in subjects with left-ventricular hypertrophy. *Circulation*. 1994;90:1786–1793.

6. Francis GS, Benedict C, Johnstone DE, et al. Comparison of neuroendocrine activation in patients with left-ventricular dysfunction with and without congestive heart failure. A substudy of the Studies of Left-Ventricular Dysfunction (SOLVD). *Circulation*. 1990;82:1724–1729.

7. Effect of enalapril on mortality and the development of heart failure in asymptomatic patients with reduced left-ventricular ejection fractions. The SOLVD investigators. *N Engl J Med*. 1992;327:685–691.

8. Kober L, Torp-Pedersen C, Carlsen JE, et al. A clinical trial of the angiotensin-converting-enzyme inhibitor trandolapril in patients with left-ventricular

dysfunction after myocardial infarction. Trandolapril Cardiac Evaluation (TRACE) study group. *N Engl J Med.* 1995;333:1670–1676.

9. Pfeffer MA, Braunwald E, Moye LA, et al. Effect of captopril on mortality and morbidity in patients with left-ventricular dysfunction after myocardial infarction. Results of the Survival and Ventricular Enlargement trial. The SAVE investigators. *N Engl J Med.* 1992;327:669–677.

10. Jong P, Yusuf S, Rousseau MF, Ahn SA, Bangdiwala SI. Effect of enalapril on 12-year survival and life expectancy in patients with left-ventricular systolic dysfunction: a follow-up study. *Lancet.* 2003;361:1843–1848.

11. Swedberg K, Held P, Kjekshus J, Rasmussen K, Ryden L, Wedel H. Effects of the early administration of enalapril on mortality in patients with acute myocardial infarction. Results of the cooperative new Scandinavian Enalapril Survival Study II (CONSENSUS II). *N Engl J Med.* 1992;327:678–684.

12. Indications for ace inhibitors in the early treatment of acute myocardial infarction: Systematic overview of individual data from 100,000 patients in randomized trials. ACE inhibitor myocardial infarction collaborative group. *Circulation.* 1998;97:2202–2212.

13. Flather MD, Yusuf S, Kober L, et al. Long-term ace-inhibitor therapy in patients with heart failure or left-ventricular dysfunction: A systematic overview of data from individual patients. ACE-inhibitor myocardial infarction collaborative group. *Lancet.* 2000;355:1575–1581.

14. Pfeffer MA, McMurray JJ, Velazquez EJ, et al. Valsartan, captopril, or both in myocardial infarction complicated by heart failure, left-ventricular dysfunction, or both. *N Engl J Med.* 2003;349:1893–1906.

15. Dargie HJ. Effect of carvedilol on outcome after myocardial infarction in patients with left-ventricular dysfunction: The CAPRICORN randomised trial. *Lancet.* 2001;357:1385–1390.

16. Chen ZM, Pan HC, Chen YP, et al. Early intravenous then oral metoprolol in 45,852 patients with acute myocardial infarction: randomised placebo-controlled trial. *Lancet.* 2005;366:1622–1632.

17. Klingbeil AU, Schneider M, Martus P, Messerli FH, Schmieder RE. A meta-analysis of the effects of treatment on left-ventricular mass in essential hypertension. *Am J Med.* 2003;115:41–46.

18. Liebson PR, Grandits GA, Dianzumba S, et al. Comparison of five antihypertensive monotherapies and placebo for change in left-ventricular mass in patients receiving nutritional-hygienic therapy in the Treatment of Mild Hypertension Study (TOMHS). *Circulation.* 1995;91:698–706.

19. Dahlof B, Devereux RB, Kjeldsen SE, et al. Cardiovascular morbidity and mortality in the Losartan Intervention For Endpoint Reduction in Hypertension Study (LIFE): A randomised trial against atenolol. *Lancet.* 2002;359:995–1003.

Chapter 8

Management of New-Onset Symptomatic Heart Failure

Key Points

- Early manifestations of symptomatic heart failure are often mistaken for other common clinical syndromes.
- Typical physical findings of congestion are often absent at the time of clinical presentation.
- High index of suspicion in at-risk patients and recognition of atypical presentations leads to faster and more accurate diagnosis.
- Recognition of symptoms is critical for appropriate treatment strategy.

Clinical Assessment

Presenting symptoms of heart failure are listed in Chapter 1. Dyspnea on exertion, orthopnea, and paroxysmal nocturnal dyspnea are the most common initial complaints of the heart failure syndrome. When a patient complains of this triad, a diagnosis of heart failure should be suspected until proven otherwise. However, it is only a minority of patients who present with this prototypical triad. Accordingly, the astute clinician must be aware of other, less typical but nonetheless common, presentations of symptomatic heart failure. If a diagnosis of heart failure is suspected, is important to obtain a detailed history for known risk factors for heart failure (Chapter 2), inflammatory diseases, genetic diseases, and exposure to cardiotoxins.

Progressive cough (usually non-productive, or mildly productive of white sputum), which persists over weeks or months, is often not recognized as a heart failure symptom and is treated with antibiotics and/or bronchodilators. The cough of early heart failure can occur in severe paroxysms associated with vomiting, and is often worse at night when the patient is supine in bed. Rales may be present on physical examination, but decreased bronchial breath sounds, or occasionally mild wheezing, is the more common finding on lung exam. If a cough thought to be due to an upper respiratory infection does not dissipate in seven to 10 days, especially in a patient with no history of lung disease or despite a course of antibiotic therapy, a careful examination for other signs of congestion such elevation of jugular venous pressures, or a gallop rhythm on cardiac exam, can be important clues to the diagnosis of heart failure (and are also linked to prognosis).[1] A chest X-ray is often useful in this setting for further evaluation of the lung parenchyma, pulmonary vasculature, and cardiac size. Evidence of cardiomegaly and/or pulmonary vascular congestion supports a diagnosis of heart failure, but absence of changes consistent with air trapping or consolidation are also important negative findings. Twelve-lead electrocardiogram and brain natriuretic peptide level are also useful screening tests to further evaluate for heart failure as a potential cause of the cough.

Abdominal bloating and/or right upper-quadrant discomfort is another common atypical presentation of heart failure that often elicits comprehensive workups for biliary disease or other gastrointestinal disorders. These symptoms are often associated with anorexia or early satiety, and if prolonged, substantial weight loss. Physical examination will often reveal an enlarged and sometimes pulsatile liver edge that may be tender to the touch. Elevated liver enzymes, hyperbilirubinemia, and hypoalbuminemia are common laboratory findings. Ultrasound imaging of the liver will generally reveal mild hepatomegaly, normal biliary tree, and a dilated inferior vena cava. Serological tests for hepatitis are negative. This cluster of findings should raise suspicions of underlying heart failure as the cause of symptoms. Physical examination for other signs of congestion (especially elevated jugular venous pressures and hepatojugular reflux), chest X-ray, 12-lead electrocardiogram, and brain natriuretic peptide level are clinically useful screening tests to confirm the diagnosis in this setting.

Patients who present with new onset of heart failure in the setting of an acute myocardial infarction represent a special subgroup of patients who may benefit from urgent coronary revascularization and other treatment strategies unique to the clinical setting of acute coronary syndromes. Detailed discussion of the evaluation and management of this subgroup is provided in Chapter 11.

While increased recognition of atypical presentations of heart failure can aid in diagnosis, it is equally important to recognize that all the signs and symptoms of heart failure (except perhaps an S3 gallop on cardiac auscultation), are non-specific and therefore may be due to non-cardiac causes.[2–4] Chronic kidney disease, a common comorbidity of patients with heart failure, is associated with sodium and water-retention and the same constellation of congestive signs and symptoms as are typical of heart failure. The spectrum of obesity hypoventilation and sleep apnea syndromes can also cause marked sodium and water retention and typical signs and symptoms of congestion. If an echocardiogram demonstrates normal ejection, normal left-ventricular thickness, normal left-atrial size, and no evidence of valvular heart disease, an evaluation for lung and kidney disease as the primary cause of symptoms is warranted.

Lower-extremity edema has a broad differential diagnosis that must be considered at the time of initial clinical suspicion for heart failure (Figure 8.1).[5] The edema associated with underlying heart failure is bilateral and typically symmetrical, usually less in the morning after supine rest, and on examination exhibits pitting that is slow to resolve. In severe edema, there may be inflammatory skin changes and weeping blisters. One of the most common non-cardiac causes of lower-extremity edema is venous insufficiency. The edema related to venous insufficiency can be differentiated from cardiac edema by the characteristic skin changes and presence of visible venous varicosities, and is often asymmetrical, especially in patients with a past saphenous vein harvest procedure for coronary artery bypass grafting. Patients will usually report that the edema is much improved or completely gone in the morning after supine rest, and worsening through the day during upright posture. Nephrotic syndrome is another common cause of non-cardiac edema. The edema related to nephrotic syndrome is typically not limited to the lower extremities, and often has associated periorbital edema, especially in the morning upon arising from supine position. The edema of nephrotic syndrome is bilateral, with pitting that tends to resolve more quickly than pitting associated with cardiac edema. Other, less common, causes of edema to consider include other hypoproteinemic states due to liver disease, malabsorption or malnutrition, edema due to the effects of anti-hypertensive therapy (arteriolar vasodilating agents, most commonly described with dihydropyridine calcium channel blockers), and conditions associated with non-pitting edema (lymphedema and myxedema).

The most useful tool to differentiate cardiac vs. non-cardiac causes of edema is a careful assessment of the jugular venous pressures.[2–4] By convention, the right jugular vein is used for estimation of the venous pressure. During physical examination, a simple screening procedure for detecting elevated jugular pressure is to examine the area between the clavicle and the mandible in the upright position (90 degrees). The patient should be instructed to relax the muscles of the neck and shoulder girdle and turn their head leftward. Normal

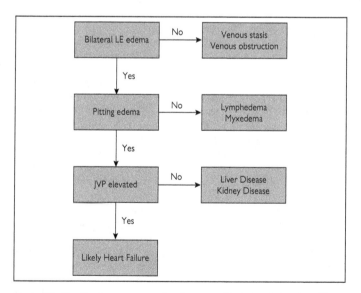

Figure 8.1 Algorithm for assessment of cardiac cause of lower extremity edema. This algorithm does not present an exhaustive differential diagnosis for edema, but highlights the more common causes of edema encountered in clinical practice. See reference 5 for full discussion of differential diagnosis of edema. For patients with likely heart failure, confirmatory testing is necessary (as described in the text) to rule out other non-cardiac diseases associated with both elevated JVP (jugular venous pressure) and edema.

jugular venous pressure waves should not be visible above the clavicle in the upright position, so the detection of waves in this position is consistent with systemic venous hypertension, most likely associated with heart failure. If the pulsations are not visible in the upright position, the patient should be reposi-tioned at 30 to 45 degrees for estimation of the height of the waves above the angle of Louis. If the pulsations are still not visible at 30 degrees, reposition the patient in the supine position. The internal jugular vein is not directly vis-ible, and its reflected waves through the subcutaneous tissues are often subtle and require time for careful inspection. The jugular venous pulsations are typi-cally seen posterior to the sternocleidomastoid muscle or near the angle of the mandible. In patients with sinus rhythm and no tricuspid regurgitation, the jugular venous pulsations have an undulating quality with two distinct compo-nents for each cardiac cycle (the "A" and "V" waves). Venous pulsations will also vary during the respiratory cycle, and may become more prominent with mild pressure over the right upper quadrant (heptojugular reflux). In patients with tricuspid regurgitation, the venous pulsation may appear to have a single component (large "V" wave), and in fact may be difficult to differentiate from the appearance of an arterial pulsation. Except in cases of extreme pulmonary hypertension, one can reliably differentiate venous pulsations and arterial pulsa-tions by simple palpation, since venous pressures are well below 60 mmHg and therefore not palpable. Suspected tricuspid regurgitation should be confirmed by the detection of a pulsatile liver edge at or below the right costal margin. In obese patients, increased subcutaneous tissue may obscure the jugular venous pulsations. There are several alternative approaches for detection of the venous pressure in this setting. The external jugular vein, which is usually seen across the mid-portion of the sternocleidomastoid muscle, although not directly con-nected to the central venous circulation can often provide an estimate of the internal jugular venous pressure. An important caveat is the recognition that the external jugular vein may contain valves that cause venous distension in the presence of normal central venous pressures. To determine if external venous distension is due to a venous valve, place one finger at the inferior portion of the vein, and use a finger on the other hand to "milk" the vein in a superior direction, so that there is no longer blood in the segment of the vein across the belly of the sternocleidomastoid muscle. While maintaining pressure of the finger in the superior position, release the finger in the inferior position and observe the vein. If the vein slowly refills from below, this observation is con-sistent with elevation of the central venous pressures. If the vein remains flat, the extended jugular vein is probably attributable to a venous valve. This can be confirmed by release of the superior finger with observation of a rapid descent of the column of blood toward the heart. This maneuver is not necessary if one can observe distinct cardiac wave pulsations in the external jugular veins. Such pulsations can only arise from the heart, so they indicate that the vein is filling due to elevated pressures in the jugular vein. Another useful technique in patients where the internal jugular venous pulsations are not easily visible due to body habitus is to carefully observe the head and neck region for other visible veins, often just superior to the sternal notch, or sometimes further pos-terior near the trapezius muscle insertion on the neck. If one can observe a vein with visible venous pulsations, these pulsations can provide a reliable estimate of jugular venous pressure. In patients with severe elevations of jugular venous pressure (>20 cm), the pressure waves may not be easily visible since they are above the angle of the mandible. In these patients, venous pulsations can often be observed at the angle of the mandible along with a bobbing earlobe, or occasionally in veins visible over the temple or the forehead. If all of the above methods fail to provide an estimate of the jugular venous pressures, inspection of the veins in the upper extremity can provide a rough estimate. An important caveat is that upper-extremity veins may become obstructed due to thrombosis in patients with frequent phlebotomies or indwelling intravenous lines. In the absence of such obstruction, a distended upper-extremity vein without thrombosis will begin to empty when the mean level of the vein is greater than the central venous pressure. The patient should be examined in the standing position, starting with hands down by the side. The dorsal veins of the hand should be distended as the hand is well below the level of the heart in this position. Ask the patient to raise the hand slowly, keeping the wrist and elbow straight. If the central venous pressure is normal, the hand veins should start to collapse as the arm achieves a position horizontal to the ground at the level of the shoulder (since this position is above the level of the right atrium). If the hand veins do not collapse until the arm is raised above the shoulder, then it is likely that the central venous pressures are elevated. If the veins do not collapse after the arm is raised above the shoulder, the veins are likely obstructed and therefore will not provide an accurate estimation of central venous pressures.

With practice, the assessment of jugular venous pressure can easily be accomplished at the bedside or office examination room in one or two minutes. Accurate estimation of the jugular venous pressure provides important information for the differential diagnosis of lower-extremity edema. Cardiac edema is invariably associated with elevation of jugular venous pressures, so the absence of elevated pressures strongly suggests a non-cardiac cause. Based on the physical examination of the edema, the estimated jugular venous pressures, and other pertinent details of the patient history, the further diagnostic evaluation for non-cardiac causes of edema can be individualized. Spot urine protein to creatinine ratio, serum albumin, and thyroid function tests are reasonable screening tests. For patients with strong suspicion of chronic venous stasis, referral for ultrasound imaging with a vascular specialist may confirm the diagnosis and also provide information relevant to treatment options.

The presence of pulmonary rales has a broad differential diagnosis that should be considered at the time of initial presentation of suspected heart failure. The rales associated with heart failure are symmetrical and typically described as fine inspiratory crackles at the bases of the lungs. If the sounds are asymmetrical or extend to the apices, other primary pulmonary causes must be considered, including pneumonia, atelectasis, and interstitial lung disease. Suspicion of a non-cardiac cause of rales is heightened by absence of other findings of congestion on exam and a low brain natriuretic peptide level. In this setting, referral to a pulmonologist for further evaluation is reasonable. As mentioned above, many patients with heart failure may not manifest typical pulmonary rales, but rather may have diffusely decreased breath sounds with a bronchial quality. Chest radiography may not be particularly useful for characterization of the cause of pulmonary rales, as evidence of pulmonary congestion is absent in a large proportion of subjects with heart failure and documented elevation of pulmonary capillary wedge pressure.[2]

Confirmatory Testing

Chest radiography and 12-lead electrocardiogram are reasonable tests to perform in all patients with suspected heart failure. The chest radiograph provides information about cardiac size and the pulmonary vasculature often clinically relevant to the differential diagnosis. Routine serial chest radiographs in patients with an established diagnosis of heart failure are not recommended. The electrocardiogram can provide information on cardiac rhythm, cardiac chamber enlargement, and evidence of conduction system disease and ischemic heart disease. Routine serial electrocardiograms are reasonable as new findings could lead to changes in therapy. A completely normal chest radiograph and electrocardiogram would reduce the level of suspicion of heart failure, but by themselves cannot rule out cardiac abnormalities associated with the heart failure syndrome.[2]

Laboratory testing—to include a comprehensive metabolic panel, complete blood count, urinalysis, and thyroid function tests—is reasonable at the initial diagnosis of heart failure. Results from these tests will not directly confirm or refute the diagnosis of heart failure, but may provide evidence of other disease processes that may exacerbate heart failure (anemia, infection, abnormal thyroid function) or contribute to the volume overload state (hypoalbuminemia, nephrotic syndrome, renal insufficiency). Since coronary artery disease is a common comorbid condition in patients with heart failure, a fasting lipid panel is also reasonable in selected patients. Additional laboratory tests to detect systemic diseases that may manifest as heart failure (iron storage studies, markers of inflammation and collagen vascular diseases), markers of infectious disease (human immunodeficiency virus [HIV] antibody, Lyme disease titer, trypanosome cruzi antibody), or infiltrative disease (serum free light chains) are reasonable in patients with suggestive clinical histories.

Brain natriuretic peptide derives its name from its original discovery in porcine brain, but in humans is predominantly a cardiac-derived peptide hormone that is secreted by cardiac muscle in response to increased stretch.[6] In cardiac muscle, this peptide hormone is initially synthesized as a long peptide chain (pre-pro-brain natriuretic peptide of 134 amino acids) and is subsequently cleaved within the myocyte to a pro-natriuretic peptide chain (108 amino acids) that is further cleaved to produce and inactive N-terminal pro-brain natriuretic peptide fragment and an active C-terminal 32-amino acid brain natriuretic peptide. Its physiological role is that of a counter-regulatory hormone to promote vasodilation and increased renal excretion of sodium in response to a volume overload state. In heart failure with symptomatic congestion, brain natriuretic peptide can be considered a failed counter-regulatory mechanism. Since synthesis of brain natriuretic peptide is increased in heart failure, measurement of both the N-terminal pro-brain natriuretic peptide fragment and the C-terminal active brain natriuretic peptide have been developed as diagnostic tests in clinical practice. Both tests perform equally well in clinical diagnostic testing, and most laboratories have selected one test or the other based on other factors related to the existing high-throughput processing systems within the laboratory. The normal ranges of the two tests differ, and the normal range of the N-terminal pro-brain natriuretic peptide fragment is age-dependent. The most clinically powerful performance characteristic of both tests is their strong negative predictive value to exclude heart failure as a cause of patient symptoms.[7] A value in the normal range is strong evidence against the presence of heart failure as a cause of symptoms of dyspnea.

One important caveat is that brain natriuretic peptide levels may be low in obese heart failure patients. Modest elevations of brain natriuretic peptide levels above the normal range may be consistent with a heart failure diagnosis based on a comprehensive assessment, but are not sufficient as the sole basis of a diagnosis of heart failure. More severe elevations (more than tenfold greater than the upper range of normal) are more likely to be associated with heart failure and are associated with poor prognosis. It is reasonable to obtain a brain natriuretic peptide level at the time of initial presentation of suspected heart failure in order to confirm the diagnosis and assist in risk stratification.

Once clinical heart failure is detected based on the history, physical examination, and laboratory evaluation as described above (with appropriate workup as necessary to exclude non-cardiac causes of edema and rales), the single most important diagnostic test is measurement of left-ventricular structure and function. Echocardiography is the most commonly used imaging modality for this purpose. The echocardiogram provides reliable information on cardiac chamber size, left-ventricular ejection fraction and regional wall motion abnormalities, cardiac valve structure and function, presence of pericardial disease, and estimates of intracardiac pressures (derived from two-dimensional images, flow Doppler and tissue Doppler measurements). Accordingly, the echocardiogram report is typically lengthy (2–3 pages) with abundant information on various aspects of the assessment. A suggested algorithm for a systematic interpretation of the information contained within the echocardiogram report is provided in Figure 8.2. The left-ventricular ejection fraction (calculated as the left-ventricular stroke volume divided by the left-ventricular end-diastolic volume) is a clinically relevant correlate of the contractile function of the heart and is a useful starting point for interpretation of the study. It is important to recognize that echocardiography is a two-dimensional imaging modality applied to the complex three-dimensional structure of the heart, and therefore is not the most accurate modality for quantitative assessment of left-ventricular ejection fraction. Keeping this caveat in mind, the estimate of left-ventricular ejection fraction from echocardiography is usually expressed as a quantitative number, with accuracy that is generally acceptable for application in clinical decision-making (with a likely estimated margin of error of ±5%). Obesity and obstructive lung disease are often associated with a substantial degradation in the quality of the ultrasound images, usually reported as a "technically difficult study." In these patients, the margin of error in the estimate of left-ventricular ejection fraction could be substantially larger. In settings where more accurate numerical assessment of ejection fraction is required, the gated radionuclide blood pool scan (MUGA scan) and cardiac MRI provide three-dimensional assessment of left-ventricular volume and highly accurate and reproducible measurement of left-ventricular ejection fraction. Based on clinical trial data, a left-ventricular ejection fraction cut-off value of ≤40% is used to identify patients with reduced systolic function who benefit from treatment strategies described below. If the left-ventricular ejection fraction is greater than 40%, other information available from the echocardiogram study can identify patients with heart failure and preserved ejection fraction. The presence of left-ventricular hypertrophy, left atrial enlargement, and/or other significant structural heart disease (moderate to severe valvular disease, abnormal shunt), and presence of elevation of the estimated pulmonary artery systolic pressure (derived from Doppler interrogation of the velocity of the tricuspid regurgitation jet) increase the likelihood of a heart failure diagnosis. The isolated presence of abnormal diastolic filling patterns detected by Doppler interrogation of mitral valve inflow in a patient with normal left-ventricular ejection fraction and no other evidence of structural heart disease is not sufficient to support a diagnosis of heart failure. Abnormal diastolic filling patterns in conjunction with elevation of the estimated pulmonary artery systolic pressure increases the likelihood of heart failure, but requires further confirmatory testing.

Testing for an assessment of coronary heart disease should also be considered for most patients with a new diagnosis of heart failure. The initial stage of testing is designed to detect the presence or absence of coronary artery disease. In a subset of patients with coronary artery disease, a second stage of testing to determine the extent of myocardial injury associated with the coronary artery disease (viability) may be indicated. The selection of the initial diagnostic test depends on the estimated risk of heart disease based on the patient's age, gender, and other known risk factors, and the patient's symptoms (presence or absence of angina). For patients with high pre-test probability of symptomatic angina, it is reasonable to consider coronary angiography as the

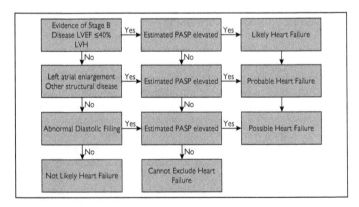

Figure 8.2 Algorithm for interpretation of echocardiogram findings in patients with new clinical diagnosis of heart failure. Echocardiographic findings must be interpreted in the context of patient symptoms and other clinical findings. An isolated finding of an abnormal diastolic filling pattern is not sufficient to make a diagnosis of heart failure. A finding of elevation of the estimated PASP (pulmonary artery systolic pressure) based on Doppler interrogation of the velocity of tricuspid regurgitation jet can be helpful to increase suspicion for heart failure.

initial test, especially if the functional capacity is severely reduced. For patients with lower pre-test probability, contraindications to an invasive procedure, or a preference to avoid an invasive procedure, non-invasive stress testing with stress perfusion imaging or stress echocardiography imaging can be performed. If possible, an exercise stress test is preferable to a pharmacological stress test. The diagnostic performance characteristics of these modalities are largely comparable but may vary by institutional expertise, so they must be individualized to each practitioner setting. Interpretation of the test results should not be limited to the presence or absence of stress-induced ischemia, but should also consider the extent of ischemic myocardium, the workload achieved, and the presence of other higher-risk findings (e.g., decrease in blood pressure, abnormal lung uptake). For patients with evidence of obstructive coronary artery disease, detected by either coronary angiography or stress testing, additional testing is often indicated to assess the potential benefits of revascularization therapy (either percutaneous or coronary artery bypass grafting). In patients with frequent angina despite optimal medical management, revascularization is effective in reducing anginal symptoms, and may be associated with a better long-term outcome. In patients without symptomatic angina, the benefits of revascularization are uncertain and must be evaluated on an individual basis.[8,9] The extent of myocardial injury (viability) can be assessed with nuclear perfusion imaging, positron emission tomography (PET) imaging, dobutamine stress echocardiography, and contrast cardiac MRI. These testing modalities assess different aspects of myocardial viability (function, anatomy, metabolism). Most existing studies suggest that any of these tests can be useful for excluding the presence of myocardial viability and therefore can be used to select patients less likely to benefit from revascularization. However, a test result consistent with viability is not closely associated with improvement in ventricular function or clinical outcomes after revascularization. Accordingly, a test result suggestive of viability should be interpreted in the clinical context: especially the degree of ventricular dysfunction (manifested as depressed left-ventricular ejection fraction) and the size of the left ventricle (left-ventricular end-diastolic dimension or volume). Patients with larger left-ventricular diastolic dimension (>6.5 cm) are less likely to derive benefit from revascularization, and were largely excluded from much of the existing literature on this topic.

A careful family history extending to all first-degree relatives should be obtained from all subjects with a new diagnosis of heart failure. A history of heart failure, heart transplantation, premature unexplained death, or cardiac disease should prompt consideration for referral to a specialized cardiovascular genetics center for further evaluation.

Right heart catheterization is not recommended as a routine assessment in all patients with new diagnosis of heart failure, but should be considered to assist in the evaluation of patients with known valvular heart disease or congenital heart disease (corrected or uncorrected), and as a gold standard test for confirmation of a heart failure diagnosis in the small subset of patients in whom the diagnosis remains uncertain despite comprehensive non-invasive evaluation.

Endomyocardial biopsy is not recommended as a routine assessment in all patients with new diagnosis of heart failure. In patients with other clinical findings suggestive of inflammatory or infiltrative disease, endomyocardial biopsy can be helpful for confirmation of diagnosis. However, endomyocardial biopsy carries greater risk than most other biopsy procedures, so it should be used only when there are no other options to confirm a tissue diagnosis of disease, and when the tissue diagnosis is likely to lead to a change in therapy for the patient.

Risk Assessment

Most patients presenting with symptomatic congestion will respond rapidly to diuretic therapy with dramatic reduction in complaints of dyspnea and improved functional capacity. Absence of a favorable response to appropriate initial therapy as discussed below suggests the patient may have some additional recognized or unrecognized comorbid condition (chronic kidney disease, nephrotic syndrome, anemia, inflammatory or infectious disease, cardiac amyloidosis, or restrictive heart disease related to past exposure to anthracycline chemotherapy or chest radiation) that limits the benefit of conventional therapy. The degree of functional capacity should be documented by assessment of the New York Heart Association Class and, in some cases, by exercise testing. This group of patients who are refractory to standard therapy requires additional diagnostic testing to identify the causes contributing to their ongoing symptoms and determine who would be likely to benefit from referral to a subspecialty heart failure tertiary center.

The assessment of left-ventricular ejection fraction and left-ventricular hypertrophy obtained from echocardiography or other imaging modalities does provide some prognostic information, but since these measures can substantially change in response to therapy, patient counseling based on these initial measures is not recommended.

Other risk assessment strategies discussed in Chapter 9 should not be performed in the early management of new onset heart failure, but rather should be delayed until the patient's treatment regimen has been optimized (optimal medical and, if indicated, surgical therapy). The rationale for this recommendation is that the large majority of patients demonstrate improvements in functional class and left-ventricular function in response to appropriate therapy. Patients should be counseled that heart failure is a serious but treatable heart condition; that it is important to continue with recommended therapies even if feeling better; and that a reassessment of their heart function in three to six months will be performed.

Treatment Strategies

The initial treatment of new onset of heart failure in most patients with congestive signs and symptoms is diuretic therapy. The class of diuretic, dosing, route, and location of this initial treatment are determined by the severity of symptoms. Patients with dyspnea at rest or minimal exertion, and patients with more than mild lower-extremity edema should be admitted to the hospital and treated with intravenous loop diuretics as described below. Patients with less severe dyspnea or minimal edema and well-preserved renal function can be treated in the outpatient setting with oral loop diuretics or thiazide diuretics with careful monitoring of electrolytes and renal function. A low threshold for hospitalization is reasonable, as the hospital location also facilitates the comprehensive evaluation described above.

For outpatients with mild symptoms, oral loop diuretics are usually first-line outpatient therapy.[10] Furosemide 20 mg daily is a reasonable starting dose for loop diuretic therapy in most patients. In patients with very mild symptoms and well-preserved renal function, a trial of thiazide diuretics is also reasonable as first-line therapy (hydrochlorothiazide 12.5 mg–25 mg daily). Patient should be advised to take their first loop diuretic dose at home or another location with easy access to restroom facilities and to start a diary of daily morning weights. The goal is to identify a dose associated with a noticeable increase in urine output within two hours of the oral dose and a gradual decrease in weight of 2–4 pounds during the first week of therapy. The dose can be titrated upwards as needed based on patient report and the weight diary. It is reasonable to provide supplemental potassium chloride 20 meq daily to prevent depletion of potassium stores (except in patients with pre-treatment serum potassium >5.0 meq/l or estimated glomerular filtration rate <30 ml/min). Electrolytes should be monitored at least weekly at the start of therapy, and quarterly once they are on a stable regimen.

For hospitalized patients with more severe symptoms, loop diuretics (most commonly furosemide, but other members of the same class, such as bumetanide and torsemide, can be substituted in equipotent doses according to Table 9.1) should be administered intravenously.[10] For a naïve patient with no past exposure to loop diuretics, an initial dose of 20 mg intravenously twice daily is reasonable. It is imperative to rapidly identify an effective diuretic dose to relieve dyspnea and other congestive symptoms. If the urine output after the initial dose is <200 cc hour over three hours, the next dose should be doubled to 40 mg (and if necessary, re-doubled to 80 mg if there is insufficient response to 40 mg). The goal is to achieve net negative fluid balance of 1–2 liters per 24 hours until symptoms are relieved and other signs of congestion are resolved (no edema, and estimated jugular venous pressure <8 cm). In patients with the anticipated large increase in urine volume and preserved renal function, potassium chloride supplements (20–40 meq twice daily) should be started to prevent depletion of potassium stores. The dose of potassium chloride should be reduced in patients with pre-treatment serum potassium >5.0 meq/l, estimated glomerular filtration rate <30 ml/min, and patients taking inhibitors of the renin-angiotensin aldosterone system. Serum electrolytes, blood urea nitrogen (BUN), and serum creatinine levels should be measured daily during intravenous loop diuretic therapy. Loop diuretics are known to induce pre-renal azotemia, so increases in blood urea nitrogen up to 50% and creatinine up to 25% over pre-treatment values are expected and not an indication to stop therapy (unless there is concomitant evidence of volume depletion manifested as hypotension with low jugular venous pressure). In patients with evidence of persistent elevation of jugular venous pressures, diuretics are unlikely to cause hypotension.

Patients who do not respond adequately to an intravenous dose of furo-semide 80 mg are considered refractory to standard diuretic therapy. Higher doses can be used (up to 200 mg intravenous furosemide twice daily), but request for consultation with a heart failure subspecialist could be considered in this setting. Evaluation for comorbid conditions that could decrease the efficacy of loop diuretics is recommended (>Stage 3 chronic kidney disease, proteinu-ria, hyperuricemia, use of corticosteroids or non-steroidal anti-inflammatory drugs). There are several strategies to overcome diuretic resistance in this set-ting. In some patients a continuous infusion of a furosemide (5–40 mg/hour) may increase total urine output over 24 hours when compared with bolus dos-ing. Disadvantages of this approach include the need for an infusion pump that may limit ability to ambulate, and possibly an increased risk of hyponatremia. An alternative approach is the addition of a thiazide diuretic (hydrochlorothi-azide 25 mg or chlorothiazide 500 mg) or thiazide-like diuretic (metolazone 2.5–5.0 mg) to the loop diuretic regimen. These two classes of diuretics act on different parts of the nephron and induce a synergistic increase in urine output. The main disadvantage of this approach is the unpredictable nature of the response, with the potential for very large increases in urine output with consequent increased risk of electrolyte depletion and hypotension. Since some patients may experience a marked increase in urine output with combination diuretic therapy, a single dose of the thiazide diuretic (rather than daily dosing) should be ordered until the response has been assessed. These thiazide diuret-ics are long-acting, so most patients do not require daily dosing.[10] Based on the response in each individual patient, dosing can be adjusted to one to three times weekly. Combination diuretic therapy is associated with substantial renal electrolyte loss, so increased potassium chloride supplements should be admin-istered, except in patients with pre-treatment serum potassium >5.0 meq/l, esti-mated glomerular filtration rate <30 ml/min, and patients taking inhibitors of the renin-angiotensin aldosterone system. It is reasonable to assess electrolytes every 12 hours during the first 48 hours of combination therapy, until a suitable potassium chloride regimen has been established to consistently maintain serum potassium levels between 4.1 and 5.1 meq/l. For patients refractory to combina-tion diuretic therapy, ultrafiltration therapy has been shown to be a safe and effective means to reduce congestion in patients with heart failure. Specialized ultrafiltration equipment for heart failure patients has been developed but may not be available at all centers. Conventional venous-venous ultrafiltration with dialysis equipment can also be used for volume removal.

Intravenous vasodilator therapy can also be considered in the initial treat-ment of hospitalized patients with new onset of heart failure and systolic blood pressure >120 mmHg.[11] Intravenous nitroglycerin is the most commonly used agent in this setting. This agent has a very short half-life, so it can be rapidly up-titrated to clinical relief of symptoms and, if necessary, can be rapidly dis-continued in the event of hypotension. The typical target dose range of intra-venous nitroglycerin for relief of dyspnea in heart failure is 100–400 mcg/min, substantially higher than the dose range for relief of angina. The intravenous infusion can be started at 10 mcg/min and doubled at five- to ten-minute inter-vals as tolerated until the patient reports symptomatic relief. Advantages of this approach include the rapid onset of action and a good safety profile associated with nitroglycerin. Disadvantages include the need for the patient to be in an appropriate facility for frequent blood pressure monitoring, and in many patients, the rapid development of tolerance to the effects of nitroglycerin within 24 hours.[12] For patients with systolic blood pressure over 180 mmHg, additional anti-hypertensive agents will probably be needed to lower systolic blood pressure to a goal of less than 130 mmHg. In the absence of evidence of a hypertensive emergency, oral anti-hypertensive agents can be added to achieve blood pressure goals. For patient with systolic blood pressure greater than 220 mmHg and/or clinical manifestations of end-organ damage of hypertensive emergency, intravenous nitroglycerin should not be used, as selective preload reduction could lead to a precipitous fall in their cardiac output. Other intravenous vasodilators, including nitroprusside, labetalol, and clevidipine, may be used in these cases.

Once the signs and symptoms of congestion have been adequately treated, further treatment strategies are determined by the initial assessment of left-ventricular ejection fraction as measured by echocardiography or other imaging modality. Accordingly, it is important to document the type of heart failure in the medical record, using appropriate codes in the problem list and progress notes (please note that International Classification of Diseases (ICD9) codes use the older terminology of "systolic heart failure" and "diastolic heart failure"). Each progress note in the medical record should also assess patients according the staging schemes discussed in Chapter 4.

The treatment strategy for patients with heart failure and reduced ejection fraction is based on observations from multiple large, controlled trials that demonstrated improved survival with recommended therapy.[13,14] Pharmacology inhibition of the renin-angiotensin aldosterone system and the sympathetic nervous system should be started in all patients with heart failure and reduced ejection fraction before hospital discharge, or in outpatients within a month of the initial diagnosis. Angiotensin-converting enzyme inhibitors are the most well-studied renin-angiotensin aldosterone system inhibitors in these patients and should be started at a low dose once the patient is clinically stable, after resolution of dyspnea at rest and during a period of stable renal function. Based on the totality of the observations from numerous clinical trials, it appears likely that all angiotensin-converting enzyme inhibitors are associated with improved functional capacity and improved clinical outcomes in patients with heart failure. Lisinopril 2.5 mg is a reasonable starting dose for normotensive patients (5 mg daily starting dose for hypertensive patients). The dose can be slowly up-titrated as tolerated to a target of 10 mg–20 mg daily. Other angio-tensin-converting enzyme inhibitor dosing guidelines are provided in Chapter 9. Angiotensin II receptor blockers can be used in patients with intolerance of angiotensin-converting enzyme inhibitors due to cough or angioedema.[15,16] There are fewer clinical trials of this class of agents in the heart failure popu-lation, with consequent uncertainty of dose-response curves and class effect. Accordingly, the two agents that have demonstrated benefit in a clinical trial in heart failure patients are recommended (valsartan starting dose 40 mg–80 mg twice daily; target dose 160 mg twice daily, and candesartan starting dose 4 mg daily; target dose 32 mg daily). Other angiotensin II receptor blockers may also be effective, but the target dose associated with reduction of mortality has not been determined. Both angiotensin-converting enzyme inhibitors and angiotensin II receptor blockers are associated with a small rise in serum creatinine due to a reduction in glomerular filtration fraction. An increase in serum creatinine of <0.5 mg/dl can be expected and is not a contraindication to continued therapy as long as the patient is not oliguric and the creatinine plateaus at this higher level. Hyperkalemia can also occur during treatment with both classes of agents. Electrolytes, blood urea nitrogen and serum creatinine levels should be closely monitored when initiating therapy or changing dose. A beta-adrenergic receptor antagonist should be added to the medical regimen once it is established that the patient is stable on a low dose of an angiotensin-converting enzyme inhibitor. Beta-adrenergic receptor blockers are a heterogenous class with clinically important differences in receptor specificity, lipophilicity, and intrinsic sympathomimetic activity. Three beta-adrenergic receptor blockers have been evaluated in clinical trials in heart failure with reduced ejection fraction: carvedilol, extended release metoprolol succinate, and bisoprolol. When compared with placebo, each of these agents was associated with substantial reduction in mortality when added to treatment with diuretics and angiotensin-converting enzyme inhibitors. These agents should be started at low dose and slowly up-titrated as tolerated to the target dose as described in Chapter 9. There is evidence of greater benefit at the highest tolerated dose, so it is important to attempt progressive up-titration to the target dose unless the patient encounters a specific intolerance. Although beta-adrenergic receptor blocking agents are used as anti-hypertensive agents in patients with high blood pressure, clinical trials have demonstrated that long-term beta-adrenergic blocker use in heart failure is actually associated with a slight increase in blood pressure compared with placebo. There is no universal blood pressure value to exclude attempted initiation of an approved beta-adrenergic receptor blocker in heart failure. Risk of symptomatic hypotension is greater in patients with systolic blood pressure <100 mmHg. Mild postural hypotension is a common side effect of this class and should not be considered a contraindication to up-titration if the resting systolic blood pressure is <100 mmHg. Beta-adrenergic receptor blockers are associated with reduction in heart rate. Resting heart rate is determined primarily by parasympathetic (vagal) tone, whereas exercise heart rate is determined primarily by sympathetic (adrenergic) tone. Accordingly, assessment of exercise heart rate rather than resting heart rate is the best approach for determination of the adequacy of beta-adrenergic receptor blockade. For patients with a resting heart rate under 60 beats/min, the patient should be asked to perform a short bout of submaximal exercise (walking in a hallway for a few minutes, or stepping on/off the step stool at the end of the office examination table for one minute [to simulate two flights of stairs]) with determination of heart rate immediately after exercise. If the heart rate increases to over 80 beats/min (and the patient is asymptomatic with systolic blood pressure >100 mmHg at rest) it is reasonable to continue up-titration of the beta-adrenergic receptor blocker. In patients with symptomatic resting sinus bradycardia (or other bradycardia rhythms associated with atrioventricular block), beta-adrenergic blocker therapy should be reduced or stopped, and further investigations for underlying sinus node dysfunction or other conduction system disease should be considered. Patients with evidence of conduction system disease may be candidates for pacemaker therapy that would allow reintroduction of beta-adrenergic blocking therapy. Beta-adrenergic receptor blockade may exacerbate bronchospasm is susceptible patients, but a history of reactive airways disease is not an absolute contraindication to such therapy in patients with heart failure. Beta-adrenergic receptor blockers should be initiated and up-titrated only after the lung disease has been stabilized, ideally in combination with anti-inflammatory therapy (local corticosteroids and leukotriene-signaling inhibition) in consultation with a pulmonologist.

Since therapy with angiotensin-converting enzyme inhibitors, angiotensin II receptor blockers, and beta-adrenergic receptor antagonists are associated with reduced mortality in patients with heart failure and reduced ejection fraction, the rationale for a clinical decision not to offer this therapy to a patient (based on a history of intolerance, contraindication, or other concern) should be documented in the medical record, preferably in an enduring portion of the medical chart such as the allergies list.

Patients hospitalized for their first presentation of heart failure with reduced ejection fraction should have diuretics, angiotensin-converting enzyme inhibition, and beta-adrenergic receptor blockade initiated at low dose before hospital discharge.[17,18] For outpatients with new onset of heart failure with reduced ejection fraction, it make take several weeks of follow-up visits to initiate these three classes. The large majority of patients will demonstrate a improvement in symptoms over the first few days to weeks of therapy, but the full benefit of the neurohormonal inhibition will not be evident for an additional three to six months. Accordingly, decisions about further specific heart failure therapy (including other medications and devices) described in the next chapters should be postponed until the patient is on the optimal doses of drugs from these three classes. The therapeutic approach for patients with persistent systolic dysfunction who remain symptomatic despite this initial treatment strategy is discussed in chapters 9 and 10.

Therapy for patients with heart failure and preserved ejection fraction is not based on clinical trials in this population, but rather on empirical recommendations for diuretic use and management of comorbidities that are closely associated with the clinical manifestations of this disease (hypertension and chronic kidney disease). If present, hypertension should be treated according to published guidelines. There is no evidence of survival benefit associated with the use of angiotensin-converting enzyme inhibitors, angiotensin II receptor antagonists, or beta-adrenergic receptor antagonists in patients with preserved ejection fraction (with or without hypertension).[19] These classes of agents may be used for control of hypertension, particularly if comorbid illnesses such as coronary artery disease and chronic kidney disease are present. Most patients with hypertension and heart failure with preserved ejection fraction will require multiple medications for blood pressure control, so reaching target blood pressure (systolic blood pressure below 130 mmHg) is more important than preferential use of any single class of drug. For patients without comorbid hypertension, there is no proven role of neurohormonal antagonists. Heart rate–lowering drug classes (beta-adrenergic receptor antagonists and non-dihydropyridine calcium antagonists) have been proposed as therapy for patients with heart failure and preserved ejection fraction, but existing literature does not support routine use of these agents.

Patients hospitalized with their first episode of heart failure with preserved ejection fraction should be treated with diuretics, and if hypertensive, a combination of anti-hypertensive drugs to achieve good blood pressure control. For outpatients with new onset of heart failure with preserved ejection fraction, diuretics and blood pressure therapy can be adjusted over several weeks. Like patients with heart failure and reduced ejection fraction, the effects of an anti-hypertensive regimen may require several months to become fully manifest.

In addition to medical therapy, all patients with new-onset heart failure should receive education about lifestyle modifications to improve functional capacity, including reduction in dietary sodium intake, participation in mild to moderate aerobic exercise as tolerated (with a goal to walk for 45 minutes once daily for at least 5 days of the week), weight loss if body mass index is higher than 30 kg/m^2, smoking cessation (if applicable), self-monitoring behaviors (daily morning weights, daily check for lower-extremity edema, and recognition of recurrent heart failure symptoms and medicine side effects), and self-efficacy behaviors (self-adjustment of diuretic dose based on daily weights, adherence to medications, and seeking medical assistance when symptoms worsen or medicine side effects occur). A discussion of advance directives is also advisable, as symptomatic heart failure is associated with a high risk of recurrent hospitalization and death.

References

1. Drazner MH, Rame JE, Stevenson LW, Dries DL. Prognostic importance of elevated jugular venous pressure and a third heart sound in patients with heart failure. *N Engl J Med.* 2001;345:574–581.

2. Butman SM, Ewy GA, Standen JR, Kern KB, Hahn E. Bedside cardiovascular examination in patients with severe chronic heart failure: importance of rest or inducible jugular venous distension. *J Am Coll Cardiol.* 1993;22:968–974.

3. Chakko S, Woska D, Martinez H, et al. Clinical, radiographic, and hemodynamic correlations in chronic congestive heart failure: conflicting results may lead to inappropriate care. *Am J Med.* 1991;90:353–359.

4. Stevenson LW, Perloff JK. The limited reliability of physical signs for estimating hemodynamics in chronic heart failure. *JAMA.* 1989;261:884–888.

5. Ely JW, Osheroff JA, Chambliss ML, Ebell MH. Approach to leg edema of unclear etiology. *J Am Board Fam Med.* 2006;19:148–160.

6. de Lemos JA, McGuire DK, Drazner MH. B-type natriuretic peptide in cardiovascular disease. *Lancet.* 2003;362:316–322.

7. Cowie MR, Jourdain P, Maisel A, et al. Clinical applications of b-type natriuretic peptide (BNP) testing. *Eur Heart J.* 2003;24:1710–1718.

8. Bonow RO, Maurer G, Lee KL, et al. Myocardial viability and survival in ischemic left-ventricular dysfunction. *N Engl J Med.* 2011;364:1617–1625.

9. Velazquez EJ, Lee KL, Deja MA, et al. Coronary-artery bypass surgery in patients with left-ventricular dysfunction. *N Engl J Med.* 2011;364:1607–1616.

10. Brater DC. Diuretic therapy. *N Engl J Med.* 1998;339:387–395.

11. Publication Committee for the VMAC Investigators (Vasodilatation in the Management of Acute CHF). Intravenous nesiritide vs. nitroglycerin for treatment of decompensated congestive heart failure: A randomized controlled trial. *JAMA.* 2002;287:1531–1540.

12. Packer M, Lee WH, Kessler PD, Gottlieb SS, Medina N, Yushak M. Prevention and reversal of nitrate tolerance in patients with congestive heart failure. *N Engl J Med.* 1987;317:799–804.

13. Flather MD, Yusuf S, Kober L, et al. Long-term ace-inhibitor therapy in patients with heart failure or left-ventricular dysfunction: A systematic overview of data from individual patients. ACE-inhibitor myocardial infarction collaborative group. *Lancet.* 2000;355:1575–1581.

14. Foody JM, Farrell MH, Krumholz HM. Beta-blocker therapy in heart failure: scientific review. *JAMA.* 2002;287:883–889.

15. Granger CB, McMurray JJ, Yusuf S, et al. Effects of candesartan in patients with chronic heart failure and reduced left-ventricular systolic function intolerant to angiotensin-converting-enzyme inhibitors: the CHARM-alternative trial. *Lancet.* 2003;362:772–776.

16. Cohn JN, Tognoni G. A randomized trial of the angiotensin-receptor blocker valsartan in chronic heart failure. *N Engl J Med.* 2001;345:1667–1675.

17. Krum H, Roecker EB, Mohacsi P, et al. Effects of initiating carvedilol in patients with severe chronic heart failure: Results from the COPERNICUS study. *JAMA.* 2003;289:712–718.

18. Packer M, Fowler MB, Roecker EB, et al. Effect of carvedilol on the morbidity of patients with severe chronic heart failure: results of the carvedilol prospective randomized cumulative survival (COPERNICUS) study. *Circulation.* 2002;106:2194–2199.

19. Yamamoto K, Sakata Y, Ohtani T, Takeda Y, Mano T. Heart failure with preserved ejection fraction. *Circ J.* 2009;73:404–410.

Chapter 9

Management of Chronic Symptomatic Heart Failure

Key Points

- Functional class and signs and symptoms of congestion should be assessed at each office visit.
- Diuretic regimen should be adjusted as needed to maintain optimal volume status at each visit for all patients with heart failure.
- Neurohormonal antagonists and eligibility for device therapy should be assessed and optimized at each encounter for patients with heart failure and reduced ejection fraction.
- Anti-hypertension therapy should be assessed and optimized at each encounter for patients with heart failure and preserved ejection fraction with history of hypertension.
- Lifestyle modifications, including smoking cessation, daily low-level aerobic exercise as tolerated, and reduction in dietary sodium, should be discussed at each patient encounter.
- Education in patient self-management should be provided to all patients to enhance their adherence to medical therapy and lifestyle recommendations.

51

Clinical Assessment

After the initial presentation of symptomatic heart failure is detected clinically (as described in the last chapter), the patient is considered to have chronic symptomatic heart failure (American College of Cardiology/American Heart Association Stage C) even if initial therapy results in complete relief of symptoms and a return to an asymptomatic state. Although this classification scheme may seem counterintuitive, a patient with transient clinical symptoms of heart failure has more advanced disease than a Stage B patient who has never had symptoms, with an associated greater risk for subsequent adverse clinical outcomes. Accordingly, the content of this chapter is relevant to all patients with a history of symptomatic heart failure, regardless of their current clinical symptoms.

All patients with a history of symptomatic heart failure will require close medical monitoring for life. For patients hospitalized with new-onset heart failure (or any subsequent hospitalization for heart failure), an outpatient visit within seven days is recommended (post-hospitalization transition of care is discussed in detail in Chapter 13). The interval between subsequent outpatient visits should be determined by the individual's severity of symptoms and the need to change or monitor medications. Treated patients in New York Heart Association Class I–II heart failure should be seen at least three times annually for blood monitoring and for detection of any disease progression.

At each outpatient visit, the patient should be carefully assessed for any signs or symptoms of worsening congestion, organ hypoperfusion, and medication side effects. Patients should be carefully questioned about symptoms of fatigue or dyspnea during activities of daily living to accurately estimate their functional capacity. Patients should be specifically questioned about the number of pillows they use at night, any interim episodes of paroxysmal nocturnal dyspnea, and the presence of abdominal bloating and edema. Patients should also be questioned about other common manifestations of heart failure (including anorexia, sleep disturbance, pain), and common medication side effects (including lightheadedness, pruritis, cough, and lower-extremity muscle cramps). Patients should be asked to record a diary of their daily weights (and blood pressure if possible) and bring the diary to each visit. The diary should be reviewed to assess any trends for weight gain or loss that may be relevant to decisions about diuretic dosing or indicative of cardiac cachexia. Patients should be asked to bring their medications to each visit. Each vial should be inspected to verify the correct medication and dose (especially for extended-release metoprolol succinate, which is often erroneously substituted by short-acting metoprolol tartrate by the pharmacy) and also to determine whether the patient has been refilling prescriptions appropriately.

The physical examination should be directed towards detection of congestion with the techniques and caveats discussed in the last chapter. It is important to recognize that many patients with chronic heart failure do not manifest the prototypical signs of congestion on physical examination. A complaint of worsening dyspnea in a patient with an established diagnosis of heart failure is likely to be related to increased volume overload, even in the absence of rales or chest radiography signs of pulmonary vascular congestion. Workup for pneumonia or pulmonary embolism should be reserved for patients with other signs and symptoms compatible with an alternative diagnosis. Blood pressure and heart rate should be obtained in the seated position and standing position if the patient has symptoms of postural lightheadedness. Patients with slow resting heart rate but stable blood pressure and no symptoms should undergo a 12-lead electrocardiogram and a brief bout of light exercise to assess the degree of beta-adrenergic receptor blockade. The patient can be asked to step on and off the step at the end of the examination table 10–20 times to simulate climbing one to two flight of stairs, or walk back and forth in an office hallway for several minutes.

Confirmatory Testing

Serum electrolytes, blood urea nitrogen, and serum creatinine levels should be checked three to four times a year and when adding or changing dose of diuretics and inhibitors of the renin-angiotensin aldosterone system. Serum digoxin levels should be checked at least twice annually, or more often in a patient with deterioration in renal function. More frequent blood testing may be considered for patients with acute or chronic kidney disease or borderline hyperkalemia. Serial brain natriuretic peptide testing is not routinely recommended in patients with an established diagnosis of chronic heart failure. Brain natriuretic peptide testing can be considered in settings where volume status is uncertain. A low value of brain natriuretic peptide suggests that the patient is currently not volume overloaded (except in obese patients), but high values do not provide a reliable assessment of the degree of volume overload. It is reasonable to routinely record a 12-lead electrocardiogram two to four times annually to assess for evidence of interim ischemia or development of an increased QRS, duration and more often for assessment of a change in symptoms, after addition of a new medication, or if there is evidence of arrhythmia on physical examination. Chest radiography should not be repeated routinely, but it can be performed as part of the assessment of a change in symptoms or to evaluate suspected lung pathology. There is no role for routine serial echocardiograms in patients with an established diagnosis of heart failure. It is reasonable to repeat echocardiograms to evaluate response to change in medical regimen, or to evaluate worsening functional capacity or other change in symptoms.

Risk Assessment

Once treatment has been optimized after the initial diagnosis of symptomatic heart failure, a repeat echocardiogram (or alternatively gated radionuclide blood pool scan or cardiac MRI) should be obtained to assess the effects of therapy on left-ventricular structure and function. For patients with heart failure with reduced ejection fraction, neurohormonal inhibition therapy may be associated with substantial increase in left-ventricular ejection fraction. Further treatment strategies discussed below are determined by the left-ventricular ejection fraction on optimal medical therapy. If the ejection fraction increases to >40% in response to neurohormonal therapy, the patient is still considered to have heart failure with reduced ejection fraction (Stage C), as the ejection fraction would probably return to pre-treatment levels if therapy were stopped. However, from the standpoint of treatment strategies discussed below, a patient with recovery of left-ventricular ejection fraction to a value >40% with well-preserved functional capacity would not require the routine administration of additional medications, or device therapy. For patients with heart failure associated with preserved ejection fraction, assessment of ventricular structure and function on optimal therapy is reasonable, although changes in ejection fraction are not expected. Effective blood pressure lowering may be associated with regression of left-ventricular hypertrophy. Other changes of chamber size, estimations of intracardiac filling pressures, and valve function may assist in further optimization of therapy.

Exercise testing after optimization of therapy may be considered on an individualized basis if clinical assessment of functional class is uncertain, since objective assessment of exercise capacity may have an impact on treatment strategies (for example, to document that a patient with heart failure and reduced ejection fraction has achieved New York Heart Association functional Class I and therefore may not be a candidate for certain additional medications and devices as described below).[1] Objective assessment of exercise capacity may also be considered in younger patients (under 60 years of age) who may be potential candidates for cardiac transplantation evaluation and patients with comorbid lung disease in whom the primary limitation of exercise capacity cannot be determined by history alone. If available, a cardiopulmonary exercise test is the recommended procedure, as the analysis of expired gases provides a quantitative assessment of peak aerobic capacity and permits differentiation of cardiac vs. pulmonary disease limitation to exercise. If cardiopulmonary exercise testing is not available, a conventional treadmill exercise test can be used to estimate peak aerobic capacity (based on metabolic equivalents), but it cannot distinguish between cardiac vs. pulmonary limitation to exercise. Routine repeat exercise stress testing is not recommended, but it can be considered at annual intervals in patients being considered for cardiac transplantation referral, or for a change in symptoms in a patient with mixed cardiopulmonary disease.

Numerous biomarkers (including brain natriuretic peptide, galectin-3, and pro-inflammatory cytokines such as tumor necrosis factor alpha) have been shown to be associated with increased risk of adverse outcomes in patients with heart failure, but the clinical utility of these blood tests has not been determined.[2] Until more evidence becomes available, these biomarkers need not be routinely obtained in clinical management. Other biomarkers, such as serum sodium, blood urea nitrogen, and hemoglobin level, are readily available for routine laboratory testing. Even mild degrees of hyponatremia, pre-renal azotemia, and anemia are associated with greater risk of mortality in patients with chronic symptomatic heart failure.

The Seattle Heart Failure Model is a prognostic risk score developed for symptomatic patients with heart failure and reduced ejection fraction.[3] The score is based on clinical data derived from demographics, physical examination, imaging and laboratory results, and medical therapies. The estimated one-year and five-year mortality risk for a patient can be easily calculated on a website sponsored by the University of Washington. The website also provides instantaneous recalculation of the one-year and five-year risk of mortality based on the addition of new medical or device therapy. Calculation of this score is not routinely recommended for all patients with heart failure and reduced ejection fraction, but it may be considered on an individual basis to aid in clinical decision-making regarding the addition of new medical therapy, implantation of an implantable cardiovertor defibrillator, or referral to a cardiac transplantation or ventricular-assist device program.

Recurrent hospitalization for heart failure in a patient with an established diagnosis of heart failure receiving optimal treatment is associated with a greatly increased risk of future rehospitalization and death.[4] Even if a specific cause of the heart failure decompensation is identified, any hospitalization event should trigger a reevaluation of the treatment regimen in order to optimize the patient's therapy and reduce the risk of subsequent adverse outcomes.

Treatment Strategies

The treatment goal in the management of chronic symptomatic heart failure is to apply the information acquired from history, physical examination, imaging, and laboratory results in order to optimize the treatment regimen for each patient.

The diuretic regimen should be reevaluated at each office visit with the goal of identifying the lowest dose of diuretics that maintains a stable optimal volume status. "Optimal volume status" is defined as absence of signs of congestion on physical examination (jugular venous pressure <8 cm of water, absence of rales, absence of lower-extremity edema [in patients without chronic venous stasis disease or other non-cardiac causes of edema]). The strategies for adjustment of diuretic regimen are based on the concept of overcoming the pharmacokinetic and pharmacodynamics factors that limit the effectiveness of diuretic therapy in patients with heart failure.[5] Furosemide is the most commonly used loop diuretic, but other loop diuretics may also be used according to the same strategies, as discussed below (Table 9.1). Signs and symptoms of increasing congestion should prompt a discussion of dietary sodium intake and counseling on the reduction of dietary sodium intake if necessary, and may require an increased dose of diuretics. The patient should be questioned carefully regarding the time(s) of day that diuretics are taken, and whether a large increase in urine output is noticeable after the dose. An effective diuretic dose should induce a large increase in urine output over several hours, with two to four episodes of spontaneous urination. If a lesser response is reported, the patient may have already achieved optimal volume status (with concomitant improvement in symptoms, stable body weight, and absence of congestion on exam), or the patient may have become resistant to their current dose of diuretic (with concomitant increased dyspnea, increased body weight, and increased congestion on physical examination). If the patient has achieved optimal volume status, cautious down-titration of the dose interval (decreasing from twice daily to once daily, or from once daily to every other day) is reasonable with instruction to maintain a diary of daily weights and return to the previous regimen if a weight gain more than three pounds is observed. If the patient's weight and clinical status remain stable, a standing diuretic regimen can eventually be substituted with an as-needed regimen based on daily weight. Down-titration of diuretics should only be attempted in stable patients (those without evidence of congestion on physical examination, and no hospitalization for heart failure within the past year) who are highly motivated to perform daily weights and who demonstrate appropriate knowledge and insight for correct interpretation and appropriate actions in response to weight change.

On the other hand, if the patient demonstrates worsening volume overload in the setting of reduced urine output response to diuretic, the dose of the diuretic (not the frequency of dosing) should be doubled with close follow-up to assess their response to the higher dose (maximum recommended single dose of furosemide is 200 mg). If the patient responds to the higher dose with resolution of volume overload, it is reasonable to attempt to down-titrate the dose based on daily weights as described above. If maximal once-daily dosing

Table 9.1 Diuretic oral dosing guidelines

Medication	Initial dose (mg)	Maximum dose (mg)	Frequency
Loop Diuretics			
Furosemide	20–40	200	QD-BID
Bumetinide	0.5–1.0	5	QD-BID
Torsemide	10–20	100	QD-BID
Thiazide diuretics			
HCTZ	25	100	QD to Q7d
Metolazone	2.5	10	QD to Q7d

does not adequately increase urine output, increased frequency of dosing is not an effective strategy. Instead, a thiazide diuretic should be cautiously added to the loop diuretic regimen, with instructions to take a single dose of the thiazide and report the urine output and weight in 24 hours. Electrolytes should be measured frequently at the initiation of combined diuretic therapy, with adjustment of potassium chloride supplements as necessary.

Some patients with worsening volume overload may report a good increase in urine output to the current dose of loop diuretic. If the history is accurate, the most likely explanation is that the dietary sodium load is very high. If the patient is not able to adhere to a lower sodium diet, it is reasonably to add a second daily dose of loop diuretic to the regimen. Since high sodium intake will increase sodium potassium exchange in the distal nephron, these patients typically require high doses of supplemental potassium chloride. Addition of a thiazide diuretic in this setting brings a higher risk of hypokalemia, so daily monitoring of serum electrolytes and adjustment of oral potassium supplementation is recommended. These patients often benefit from addition of spironolactone to the regimen. Serum potassium levels must be measured frequently at initiation of therapy with the expectation that the potassium chloride supplement requirements will decrease.

Changes in volume status and diuretic responsiveness in patients with chronic heart failure are often associated with concomitant changes in renal function. In many cases, the primary cause of these changes is not easily discernible, due to a complex interplay between the effects of volume overload, renal perfusion, diuretics, and neurohormonal antagonists on the glomerular filtration rate. In the setting of worsening dyspnea with clear signs of volume overload on physical examination (including elevation of the jugular venous pressure), it is reasonable to increase the diuretic dose to relieve patient symptoms. As the jugular vein pressure decreases in response to effective diuretic therapy, renal function will often spontaneously improve. However, if pre-renal azotemia worsens in response to increased diuretic therapy, further adjustment of diuretics should be based on a careful assessment for signs of low cardiac output (hypotension, narrow pulse pressure, thready pulse or pulsus alternans, cool extremities). For patients who appear to remain well perfused despite worsening azotemia, diuretic therapy should be continued to maintain optimal volume status. Many of these patients have comorbid chronic kidney disease and benefit from multidisciplinary management, as described in

Chapter 11. Available evidence suggests that the elimination of congestion is associated with improved clinical outcomes, even in the setting of worsening renal function.[6-8] For patients with evidence of persistent congestion, worsening renal function, and systemic hypoperfusion, hospitalization should be considered ("cold and wet"; see further discussion in Chapter 12). This constellation of signs and symptoms is associated with high mortality risk and should prompt discussion of advance directives and patient eligibility for advanced therapies (see further discussion in Chapter 10).

For patients with worsening azotemia in the absence of signs and symptoms of volume overload, it is reasonable to temporarily reduce or discontinue diuretics, and monitor daily weights and symptoms. If the volume status is uncertain due to contradictory information (for example, worsening dyspnea without increased weight or clear evidence of worsening congestion on exam), additional assessment (chest radiograph, brain natriuretic peptide level, and/or right-heart catheterization) should be obtained to guide therapy.

For patients with heart failure with reduced ejection fraction, neurohormonal-antagonist therapy should be reviewed and optimized at each visit with the goal of achieving the maximum tolerated target dose of each class of agent (Tables 9.2 and 9.3). After establishing the initial diagnosis, low doses of both angiotensin-converting enzyme inhibitors (or, if intolerant due to cough or angioedema, angiotensin-receptor blockers) and beta-adrenergic receptor blockers should be initiated as described in the last chapter. A strategy for optimizing the doses of neurohormonal antagonists is summarized in Figure 9.1.

At each subsequent outpatient visit, the dose of the beta-adrenergic receptor blocker should be doubled as tolerated to achieve the target dose known to be associated with reduced mortality risk (Table 9.3).[9] Mild orthostatic hypotension symptoms can be expected during up-titration and do not constitute contraindication of further up-titration of dose. Postural symptoms tend to wane during long-term therapy. Blood pressure may transiently decrease during up-titration of therapy, but it tends to return to baseline over time. Systolic blood pressure >90 mmHg is acceptable as long as the patient is asymptomatic. Reduction in resting heart rate is also to be expected. Heart rate less than 60 bpm is not a contraindication to further up-titration unless there is evidence of greater than first-degree atrioventricular block, symptomatic hypotension, or failure to increase heart rate to >80 beats per minute with mild exercise. Patients with severe chronotropic incompetence on a low dose of beta-adrenergic receptor blocker should be evaluated for evidence of intrinsic conduction system disease, with consideration for placement of permanent pacemaker therapy as necessary. Patients receiving amiodarone are more likely to manifest bradyarrhythmias during up-titration of beta-adrenergic receptor blockers, but the same principles can be applied for up-titration. Diuretic dosing should be reevaluated after completion of titration, as many patients on stable maximal tolerated target doses of beta-adrenergic blockers will require lower doses of diuretics to maintain optimal volume status.

Once the highest tolerated target dose of the beta-adrenergic receptor blocker has been achieved, the angiotensin-converting enzyme inhibitor (or angiotensin-receptor blocker) should be advanced to target doses as tolerated (Table 9.2).[10] A small increase in creatinine of 0.1–0.5 mg/dl is expected in

Table 9.2 Dosing guidelines for inhibitors of the renin-angiotensin aldosterone system in heart failure with reduced ejection fraction. All of the agents listed in this table share common side effects of hypotension, worsening renal function, and hyperkalemia. The risk of these side effects is increased when these agents are used in combination. Patients with comorbid chronic kidney disease (estimated glomerular filtration rate <30 ml/min) are at greater risk for these side effects. In this population, lower doses and more frequent monitoring should be used to reduce risk

Medication	Initial Dose (mg)	Target Dose (mg)	Frequency
Angiotensin-converting enzyme inhibitors			
Captopril	6.25	50	TID
Enalapril	2.5–5	10–20	BID
Lisinopril	2.5–5	20–40	QD
Ramipril	1.25–2.5	5	BID
Trandolapril	1	4	QD
Quinapril*	5	20	BID
Fosinopril*	5–10	40	QD
Angiotensin-Receptor Blockers (as alternative to ACE inhibitor)			
Candesartan	4	32	QD
Valsartan	40	160	BID
Losartan†	25	150	QD
Mineralocorticoid receptor antagonists			
Spironolactone	25	50	QD
Eplerenone	25	50	QD

* indicates that these agents are approved by the Food and Drug Administration (FDA) for heart failure but have not been shown to reduce morbidity and mortality in heart failure.

† indicates that this agent is not FDA-approved for heart failure. Dose recommendation is based on data from reference 13.

Table 9.3 Dosing recommendation for beta-adrenergic receptor blockers for patients with heart failure with reduced ejection fraction. Other beta-adrenergic blockers (including short-acting metoprolol tartrate) have not been proven to reduce risk of adverse outcomes in patients with heart failure with reduced ejection fraction

Medication	Initial Dose (mg)	Target Dose (mg)	Frequency
Metoprolol Succinate (extended release)	25	200	QD
Carvedilol	3.125	25	BID
Bisoprolol*	2.5	10	QD

*Bisoprolol has been shown to reduce risk of adverse outcomes when compared with placebo, but is not approved in the United States for a heart failure indication.

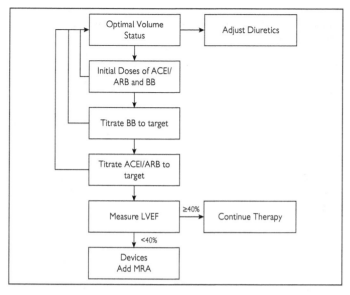

Figure 9.1 Strategy for optimization of therapy for patients with heart failure and reduced ejection fraction.

response to angiotensin-converting enzyme inhibitor or angiotensin-receptor blocker therapy. If the patient is non-oliguric, and the creatinine plateaus during therapy, therapy can be up-titrated with continued careful monitoring. Cough is a well-known side effect of angiotensin-converting enzyme inhibitors, but it is also a common symptom of heart failure. The cough associated with heart failure is often productive of scant white sputum and occurs most often at night or early morning upon arising. The cough associated with angiotensin-converting enzyme inhibitors is typically non-productive, occurs intermittently throughout the day (less so at night), and is often triggered by speaking, or drinking cold fluids. A complaint of cough should prompt a careful assessment for evidence of worsening congestion or comorbid lung disease. In the absence of evidence of worsening congestion, it is reasonable to switch from an angiotensin-converting enzyme inhibitor to a comparable dose of an angiotensin-receptor blocker (based on the percentage of target dose for each agent, per Table 9.2). If the cough is due to the angiotensin-converting enzyme inhibitor, the patient will usually notice substantial reduction in cough within one week of cessation of the drug. Candesartan and valsartan have been shown to reduce the risk of adverse clinical outcomes in patients with heart failure with reduced ejection fraction intolerant of angiotensin converting enzyme inhibitors and are approved for this indication.[11,12] Due to pharmacy formulary limitations, many patients do not have access to all available angiotensin-receptor blockers. Losartan, although not approved for heart failure, is the most widely available and has been shown to reduce risk of adverse outcomes in heart failure patients with reduced ejection fraction at a target dose of 150 mg daily.[13] Angioedema is a less common side effect of angiotensin-converting enzyme inhibitors. Although angioedema has also been rarely described with angiotensin-receptor blockers, it is reasonable to substitute therapy with an angiotensin-receptor blocker in patients with angioedema in response to an angiotensin-converting enzyme inhibitor, as the risk of recurrence appears to be exceedingly low.[11,12] Hypotension is another known potential side effect of both angiotensin-converting enzyme inhibitors and angiotensin-receptor blockers. For patients without ongoing signs of congestion (normal jugular venous pressure and absence of rales and edema), it is reasonable to reduce the dose of diuretics during initiation and up-titration to minimize the risk of symptomatic hypotension. Hyperkalemia may also be observed with both angiotensin-converting enzyme inhibitors and angiotensin-receptor blockers. The risk is greatest in patients with comorbid chronic kidney disease. Reduced dietary potassium (including elimination of potassium-containing salt substitutes) and more frequent laboratory monitoring can reduce the risk of symptomatic hyperkalemia in these patients.

Many patients in clinical practice settings receive doses of neurohormonal antagonists (beta-adrenergic receptor antagonists and renin-angiotensin-aldosterone system inhibitors) that are lower than those utilized in clinical trials. Titration of neurohormonal antagonists to the maximal tolerated target dose is important, as available evidence supports an important dose–response relationship for these classes of drugs. Most side effects during up-titration are transient and may not be reproducible, so if intolerance is encountered at a certain dose level, it is reasonable to make a second effort at up-titration at a later date. A systematic assessment of guideline recommended therapy at each patient encounter is a useful approach to increase the likelihood of titration to the maximal tolerated target dose.

After upward titration has been completed (typically within three to six months of initiation of therapy), functional capacity should be assessed and left-ventricular ejection fraction should be re-measured as described above. If the patient remains symptomatic with left-ventricular ejection fraction <40% after three to six months of optimal therapy, several different options should be considered. Additional medical therapy with a mineralocorticoid receptor antagonist is warranted to further relieve symptoms and reduce mortality risk (Table 9.2).[14–16] Spironolactone 25 mg–50 mg once daily or eplerenone 25 mg–50 mg once daily should be added if the estimated glomerular filtration rate is >30 ml/min and the serum potassium is <5.1 meq/l. The major risks of combined therapy of a mineralocorticoid receptor antagonist with an angiotensin-converting enzyme inhibitor or angiotensin-receptor blocker are hyperkalemia and worsening renal function. The onset of these adverse events is somewhat unpredictable but most often occurs in the first few months of therapy, so increased frequency of laboratory monitoring is required. Digoxin (0.125 mg–0.25 mg daily) can also be added to the medical regimen in this group.[17] No loading dose is required. The dose should be adjusted for renal insufficiency as needed to maintain a serum level ≤1 ng/ml.[18,19] Once the serum level is in the desired range, the level should be checked semi-annually, or more often for signs or symptoms suggestive of digitalis toxicity, or change in renal function. Combination vasodilator therapy with hydralazine and isosorbide dinitrate (starting dose, 37.5 mg hydralazine and 20 mg isosorbide dinitrate together three times daily, up-titrated to double the starting dose of each agent as tolerated) can be used as an alternative vasodilator regimen for patients intolerant of angiotensin-converting enzyme inhibitors and angiotensin-receptor blockers due to worsening renal function, and can also be added in the subgroup of patients self-identified as African-American.[20,21] This vasodilator combination has been shown to substantially reduce mortality risk in this group, but application in clinical practice is limited by difficulty in adherence to the three-times-daily dosing regimen, and common side effects of lightheadedness and headache. Patients treated with nitrates should not take phosphodiesterase type 5 inhibitors for erectile dysfunction (sildenafil, vardenifil, tadalafil) due to the risk of a dangerous drop in blood pressure.

Routine oral anticoagulation therapy with warfarin is not recommended for patients with heart failure with reduced ejection fraction in normal sinus rhythm.[22] Chronic oral anticoagulation therapy with warfarin is recommended for patients with atrial fibrillation, patients with mobile intracardiac thrombi, or a previous history of arterial or venous thromboembolic events. Low-dose aspirin (81 mg) can be safely administered to patients with heart failure and history of remote myocardial infarction or past stroke or transient ischemic attack (TIA). There is no proven role for routine use of aspirin for patients without a history of myocardial infarction or stroke, so the treatment must be individualized based on the risk of thrombotic events.

Patients with persistent symptoms and reduced left-ventricular ejection fraction (≤35%) on optimal medical therapy should also be evaluated for implantation of a cardiovertor defibrillator device to reduce the risk of sudden death.[23,24] In the subpopulation of patients with reduced left-ventricular ejection fraction and evidence of intraventricular conduction delay on the electrocardiogram (left bundle branch block or other morphology with QRS duration >150 msec), a combined biventricular resynchronization pacemaker and implantable cardiovertor defibrillator is recommended.[25]

Patients with heart failure and reduced ejection fraction often elect to take nutritional supplements such as L-carnitine and coenzyme Q-10. There are very few controlled prospective studies with unbiased evaluation of the clinical efficacy of these agents. These "natural" remedies may provide a sense of control for patients and thus may indirectly contribute to a stronger sense of self-management that can be beneficial for the overall treatment plan. Accordingly, it is recommended to document the use of supplements taken by the patient with surveillance to exclude any supplements with known potential harm (sympathomimetics).

For patients with an initial diagnosis of heart failure with reduced ejection fraction who, on optimal therapy with angiotensin-converting enzyme inhibitor and beta-adrenergic receptor blocker, demonstrate an increase in ejection fraction to >40%, or who have returned to normal functional capacity (New York Heart Association Class I), the additional medical and device therapies discussed in the preceding paragraphs are not routinely recommended, but may be considered on an individualized basis.

For patients with initial diagnosis of heart failure with preserved ejection fraction, the diuretic regimen should be optimized as discussed above. In the subgroup with hypertension, the hypertension regimen should be optimized at each visit to achieve blood pressure goals with minimization of side effects. Older hypertensive patients often present with isolated systolic hypertension (with associated large pulse pressure). This clinical entity is attributable to increased aortic stiffness, with consequent increased pulse wave velocity and increased hydraulic load on the left ventricle during systole. The increased stiffness in the aorta is primarily attributable to loss of the elastic components in the blood vessel wall. Currently available anti-hypertensive therapies do not directly impact the elasticity in the aorta, so anti-hypertensive therapy typically reduces both systolic and diastolic blood pressures with little change in pulse pressure. In patients with coronary artery disease, excessive reduction in diastolic blood pressure can compromise myocardial blood flow during diastole and induce ischemia. Therapy must be individualized based on the perceived risks of myocardial ischemia, with a goal to keep diastolic blood pressure >65 mmHg.

All patients with chronic symptomatic heart failure should receive ongoing education in lifestyle modifications to improve their quality of life, including reduction in dietary sodium, participation in moderate aerobic exercise activities as tolerated, and relevant self-monitoring and self-efficacy behaviors as described in Chapter 13. Physical training has been shown to be safe and associated with improved functional capacity in patients with heart failure with both preserved and reduced ejection fraction. Referral to an outpatient cardiac rehabilitation program should be considered for motivated individuals; however, most medical insurance will not provide coverage for outpatient therapy unless there is comorbid coronary artery disease.

Erectile dysfunction occurs commonly in men with chronic heart failure. Sildenafil at doses ranging from 25 mg–100 mg daily has been shown to be well tolerated in patients with heart failure with functional capacity that permits sexual activity.[26] Sildenafil and related agents should not be administered to patients treated with organic nitrates due to risk of hypotension. These agents should also be used with caution in patients taking alpha-adrenergic receptor blockers for treatment of prostatic hypertrophy.

Most patients with chronic heart failure respond well to optimal medical treatment, with reduction in congestive signs and symptoms and improved functional capacity. These patients should be followed within the practice setting of the primary care provider and/or cardiologist at three- to six-month intervals as determined by the severity of symptoms. Patients with high-risk features (hospitalizations, multiple comorbidities) should be seen more frequently and may benefit from referral to specialized heart failure centers as described in Chapter 13.

The most carefully crafted therapeutic regimen will not provide optimal benefit to the patient who fails to reliably adhere to the prescribed regimen. Several lines of evidence indicate that the majority of patients with chronic heart failure do not fully adhere to their prescribed medical regimen. Once-daily medications and fixed-dose combination medications should be used when feasible to simplify the medical regimen. It is important to engage the patient in a non-judgemental manner to elicit barriers to full adherence, and develop plans to address these barriers. Most patients would prefer to take fewer pills and are naturally skeptical of lifelong prescriptions. Many patients are tempted to temporarily stop their medications to determine whether they can detect any difference in their well-being. Since many of the neurohormonal antagonists may be transiently stopped with no apparent change in symptoms, it is important to educate the patient about the purpose of each medication at each encounter, with emphasis on the fact that some medications are not primarily used to reduce symptoms, but rather to slow the progression of the disease (and improve their survival). A simple review of all medications at each visit, with the stated intention to find any that are no longer needed, and a brief reinforcement statement for the purpose of the medications to be continued may enhance adherence.

Medical decision-making for ambulatory heart failure patients is generally considered to be complex due to the underlying complex pathophysiology, polypharmacy, and high risk of mortality and other adverse clinical outcomes. Medical record documentation for each heart failure patient encounter should include a comprehensive assessment of typical and atypical symptoms, a detailed physical examination that includes typical and atypical signs of congestion, a comprehensive assessment that includes statement of the disease stage (per American College of Cardiology and American Heart Association guidelines), the functional class (per New York Heart Association classification), the volume status of the patient (hypovolemic, optimal, or hypervolemic), evaluation of optimization of medical and device therapy, and a statement on patient

Table 9.4 Suggested components for medical documentation for ambulatory heart failure patients

History	Exercise tolerance (number of blocks, flights)
	Orthopnea (number of pillows)
	Paroxysmal nocturnal dyspnea
	Nocturia
	Fatigue
	Sleep disturbance
	Anorexia
	Adherence
Physical Examination	Presence of cachexia
	Description of pulse volume, pulsus alternans
	Description of breathing pattern
	Estimation of jugular venous pressure
	Presence of rales or bronchial breath sounds
	Location of point of maximal impulse (PMI), presence of gallop or murmur
	Presence of hepatomegaly and ascites
	Presence of pre-sacral or lower-extremity edema
	Cool vs. warm extremities
Assessment	Type of heart failure (preserved vs. reduced ejection fraction)
	ACC/AHA Stage
	NYHA Class
	Volume status
	Evaluation of optimization of therapy
	Statement of patient education

self-management education (Table 9.4). Paper or electronic templates can be used to increase consistency in the management of this population. Incorporation of combined nursing and physician participation during patient encounters is another useful strategy for optimization of therapy and education. If these practices are not feasible for a given practice setting, referral to a specialized heart failure center should be considered.

References

1. Aaronson KD, Schwartz JS, Chen TM, Wong KL, Goin JE, Mancini DM. Development and prospective validation of a clinical index to predict survival in ambulatory patients referred for cardiac transplant evaluation. *Circulation*. 1997;95:2660–2667.

2. Braunwald E. Biomarkers in heart failure. *N Engl J Med*. 2008;358:2148–2159.

3. Levy WC, Mozaffarian D, Linker DT, et al. The Seattle Heart Failure Model: prediction of survival in heart failure. *Circulation*. 2006;113:1424–1433.

4. O'Connor CM, Abraham WT, Albert NM, et al. Predictors of mortality after discharge in patients hospitalized with heart failure: an analysis from the organized program to initiate lifesaving treatment in hospitalized patients with heart failure (optimize-HF). *Am Heart J*. 2008;156:662–673.

5. Brater DC. Diuretic therapy. *N Engl J Med*. 1998;339:387–395.

6. Drazner MH, Rame JE, Stevenson LW, Dries DL. Prognostic importance of elevated jugular venous pressure and a third heart sound in patients with heart failure. *N Engl J Med*. 2001;345:574–581.

7. Gheorghiade M, Follath F, Ponikowski P, et al. Assessing and grading congestion in acute heart failure: a scientific statement from the Acute Heart Failure Committee of the Heart Failure Association of the European Society of Cardiology and endorsed by the European Society of Intensive Care Medicine. *Eur J Heart Fail*. 2010;12:423–433.

8. Metra M, Davison B, Bettari L, et al. Is worsening renal function an ominous prognostic sign in patients with acute heart failure? The role of congestion and its interaction with renal function. *Circ. Heart Fail*. 2012;5:54–62.

9. Foody JM, Farrell MH, Krumholz HM. Beta-blocker therapy in heart failure: scientific review. *JAMA*. 2002;287:883–889.

10. Flather MD, Yusuf S, Kober L, et al. Long-term ACE-inhibitor therapy in patients with heart failure or left-ventricular dysfunction: A systematic overview of data from individual patients. ACE-Inhibitor Myocardial Infarction Collaborative Group. *Lancet*. 2000;355:1575–1581.

11. Cohn JN, Tognoni G. A randomized trial of the angiotensin-receptor blocker valsartan in chronic heart failure. *N Engl J Med*. 2001;345:1667–1675.

12. Granger CB, McMurray JJ, Yusuf S, et al. Effects of candesartan in patients with chronic heart failure and reduced left-ventricular systolic function intolerant to angiotensin-converting-enzyme inhibitors: the CHARM-alternative trial. *Lancet*. 2003;362:772–776.

13. Konstam MA, Neaton JD, Dickstein K, et al. Effects of high-dose versus low-dose losartan on clinical outcomes in patients with heart failure (HEAAL Study): A randomised, double-blind trial. *Lancet*. 2009;374:1840–1848.

14. Pitt B, Remme W, Zannad F, et al. Eplerenone, a selective aldosterone blocker, in patients with left-ventricular dysfunction after myocardial infarction. *N Engl J Med*. 2003;348:1309–1321.

15. Pitt B, Zannad F, Remme WJ, et al. The effect of spironolactone on morbidity and mortality in patients with severe heart failure. Randomized Aldactone Evaluation Study investigators. *N Engl J Med.* 1999;341:709–717.

16. Zannad F, McMurray JJ, Krum H, et al. Eplerenone in patients with systolic heart failure and mild symptoms. *N Engl J Med.* 2011;364:11–21.

17. The Digitalis Investigation Group. The effect of digoxin on mortality and morbidity in patients with heart failure. *N Engl J Med.* 1997;336:525–533.

18. Gheorghiade M, van Veldhuisen DJ, Colucci WS. Contemporary use of digoxin in the management of cardiovascular disorders. *Circulation.* 2006;113:2556–2564.

19. Smith TW. Digitalis. Mechanisms of action and clinical use. *N Engl J Med.* 1988;318:358–365.

20. Cohn JN, Archibald DG, Ziesche S, et al. Effect of vasodilator therapy on mortality in chronic congestive heart failure. Results of a Veterans Administration cooperative study. *N Engl J Med.* 1986;314:1547–1552.

21. Taylor AL, Ziesche S, Yancy C, et al. Combination of isosorbide dinitrate and hydralazine in blacks with heart failure. *N Engl J Med.* 2004;351:2049–2057.

22. Homma S, Thompson JL, Pullicino PM, et al. Warfarin and aspirin in patients with heart failure and sinus rhythm. *N Engl J Med.* 2012;366:1859–1869.

23. Bardy GH, Lee KL, Mark DB, et al. Amiodarone or an implantable cardioverter-defibrillator for congestive heart failure. *N Engl J Med.* 2005;352:225–237.

24. Moss AJ, Hall WJ, Cannom DS, et al. Improved survival with an implanted defibrillator in patients with coronary disease at high risk for ventricular arrhythmia. Multicenter Automatic Defibrillator Implantation Trial investigators. *N Engl J Med.* 1996;335:1933–1940.

25. Bristow MR, Saxon LA, Boehmer J, et al. Cardiac-resynchronization therapy with or without an implantable defibrillator in advanced chronic heart failure. *N Engl J Med.* 2004;350:2140–2150.

26. Katz SD, Parker JD, Glasser DB, et al. Efficacy and safety of sildenafil citrate in men with erectile dysfunction and chronic heart failure. *Am J Cardiol.* 2005;95:36–42.

Chapter 10

Management of Advanced Chronic Symptomatic Heart Failure

Key Points

- The characterization of advanced heart failure is determined by the functional capacity of the patient rather than the left-ventricular ejection fraction.
- Patients with severe limitation of functional capacity have a high risk of hospitalization and death, independent of ejection fraction.
- If no reversible causes of disease progression are identified, patients should be evaluated for advanced therapies (cardiac transplantation or mechanical circulatory support), or if not eligible for such therapies, for palliative care and hospice referral.
- It is reasonable to consider reduction of dose or withdrawal of neuro-hormonal antagonist therapy in patients with advanced heart failure and intolerable side effects.
- It is reasonable to consider deactivation of implantable cardiovertor defibrillators in patients with advanced heart failure and estimated survival of less than one year.
- Vasodilators and positive inotropic agents may be used acutely and chronically to alleviate symptoms in this population as part of a comprehensive palliative care program.

Clinical Assessment

The characterization of advanced heart failure (Stage D) is primarily determined by the functional capacity of the patient rather than the left-ventricular ejection fraction. Patients with advanced heart failure have poor quality of life due to severely reduced functional capacity despite optimal medical and device therapy. Simple activities of daily living such as bathing and dressing can induce severe dyspnea, often require long, frequent rests to complete the task, and leave the patient feeling exhausted. Other distressing symptoms in this group included profound fatigue, sleep disturbance, restlessness, lethargy, poor concentration, hair loss, alteration of taste sensation, sexual dysfunction, and anorexia with weight loss.

Careful questioning about symptoms during specific activities is important, as many patients slowly curtail activities that produce dyspnea or fatigue without conscious acknowledgement of their change in lifestyle, and come to accept frequent dyspnea and fatigue with minimal exertion as a "normal" aspect of their heart condition. If a severe limitation in functional capacity is detected, the patient should be further questioned about day-to-day changes in the symptoms, since patterns in the daily severity of symptoms can sometimes help determine treatment strategies. Specific questions on sleep patterns and the physical symptoms that interrupt sleep may also be helpful to identify strategies to reduce fatigue. Specific information on patterns of food intake can identify strategies to improve nutrition and stamina. Depression, chronic pain, impaired concentration, and an uncomfortable sense of restlessness are common symptoms in this stage of the disease. Specific questions on these issues are useful to identify these conditions as potential targets for palliative therapy.

On physical examination, patients with advanced heart failure often demonstrate cachexia (characterized by bitemporal wasting, wasting of the musculature of the shoulder girdle, and generalized muscle atrophy) and appear fatigued. In some cases, there may be psychomotor retardation and slowed speech. In patients with advanced heart failure and reduced ejection fraction, the pulse pressure is often narrowed, with a thready pulse or pulsus alternans evident on palpation of the radial artery.[1] Prolonged observation of respiration will often reveal a Cheyne-Stokes pattern of periodic breathing.[2] Extremities are typically cool to the touch. Signs of congestion are often present, but in many cases may be no different than the patient's baseline.

Laboratory data will often demonstrate worsening pre-renal azotemia and hyponatremia. Anemia is also more common in patients with advanced heart failure, probably due to a combination of factors that reduce red cell production and increase hemodilution.

Diuretic resistance is another clinical marker of low-cardiac-output syndrome in patients with other features of advanced heart failure. Diuretic resistance can be rapidly assessed by a spot sample for urinary sodium concentration one hour after a dose of intravenous loop diuretic. If the urinary sodium is <70 meq/l, the response to the diuretic is suboptimal. If the diuretic dose is already in excess of furosemide 80 mg (or its equivalent with other loop diuretics), other strategies including combination diuretic therapy (as discussed in chapters 8 and 9) or additional intravenous therapy to increase cardiac output and renal perfusion should be considered.

Confirmatory Testing

It is reasonable to consider a repeat echocardiogram in the setting of worsening symptoms, especially if the interval from the last study is more than 12 months, or there is clinical suspicion of an interim change in ventricular function or valve function. For patients with heart failure and reduced ejection fraction, imaging may detect an increase in the left-ventricular end-diastolic dimension from prior studies, decrease in the left-ventricular ejection fraction from prior studies, and new or worsening mitral and tricuspid regurgitation. For patients with heart failure with preserved ejection fraction, subtle changes in left-ventricular size and left-ventricular ejection fraction from the patient baseline may be present, although typically not outside of the normal range.

Many of the signs and symptoms of advanced heart failure are related to severe reductions in cardiac output reserve. Right-heart catheterization may be considered to confirm the clinical suspicion of reduced cardiac output, and also to directly measure cardiac filling pressures (to rule out volume depletion as a cause of the worsening symptoms). Estimated cardiac outputs derived from the Fick formula are more reliable than thermodilution cardiac output measurements in patients with advanced heart failure. Due to the invasive nature of this procedure, right-heart catheterization is not recommended routinely for all patients, but it should be performed in patients who may be candidates for mechanical circulatory support and/or cardiac transplantation as discussed below (age less than 75 years with no non-cardiac disabling or life-limiting conditions).

It is recommended to obtain an electrocardiogram and chest radiograph in the evaluation of a patient with worsening symptoms. Routine testing for change in coronary anatomy (stress testing and/or coronary angiography) is not recommended but can be considered in patients with relevant electrocardiographic findings or symptoms suggestive of myocardial ischemia. Elevations of serum troponin to two to three times the upper limit of normal is common in this population and is not diagnostic for acute coronary syndrome in the absence of clinical symptoms and/or electrocardiographic evidence of acute ischemia.

Risk Stratification

The severe limitation in functional capacity is the most important marker of poor outcome in this population. If a reliable history cannot be obtained, cardiopulmonary exercise testing can be performed to objectively measure peak aerobic capacity. A peak oxygen consumption <14 ml/kg/min (or less than 50% of predicted) is associated with poor outcome (<85% one-year survival).[3] For patients with advanced heart failure with reduced ejection fraction in whom the peak oxygen uptake measure is available, the Heart Failure Survival Score can be calculated to estimate one-year mortality risk.[4] In patients with advanced heart failure, many other biomarkers of poor outcome are often present (hyponatremia, worsening azotemia, elevated brain natriuretic peptide).[5] Documented unintentional weight loss (at "dry" weight) of more than 5% of body weight is a strong predictor of poor outcome in this population.[6] Biomarkers of poor nutrition (low albumin, low protein, anemia) are usually present and are also associated with increased risk of adverse outcomes.[7,8] Increased pulmonary capillary wedge pressure and other measures of elevated pulmonary vascular resistance and decreased right-ventricular function determined at the time of right-heart catheterization are also associated with poor outcome.[3,9]

Treatment Strategies

It is reasonable to consider hospitalization of patients with worsening symptoms in order to facilitate optimization of therapy (see further discussion in Chapter 12). Other sites of care, including emergency departments, outpatient furosemi-de-infusion centers, medical homes, or hospices, may be reasonable alternatives to consider in patients with advanced heart failure. Optimization of volume status should be a priority for all patients with advanced heart failure, with recognition that worsening azotemia and hypotension in response to diuretic therapy are quite common in this group. While relief of congestion is a desirable goal, patients with advanced heart failure may continue to be highly symptomatic despite optimization of volume status, due to reduced cardiac output reserve. The syndrome of low cardiac output is differentiated from cardiogenic shock by the degree of hypotension and clinical hypoperfusion of vital organs. In the low-cardiac-output syndrome there may be evidence of mild organ dysfunction, but lactic acid levels in the blood are usually normal, or only minimally elevated. Cardiogenic shock is characterized by severe multiorgan failure and lactic aci-dosis. A detailed discussion of the treatment of cardiogenic shock is beyond the scope of this book, but it is closely related to the therapeutic principles for restoration of organ perfusion as described below. Neurohormonal-inhibition treatment strategies used in earlier stages of heart failure may be poorly tolerated in patients with advanced heart failure. In patients with reduced ejection fraction, hypotension and worsening renal function may necessitate down-titration or withdrawal of inhibitors of the renin-angiotensin aldosterone system and sympathetic nervous system.

Patients with reduced ejection fraction and the clinical syndrome of low-cardiac-output syndrome (determined either clinically or on the basis of right-heart catheterization data) will usually derive symptomatic relief with treatment directed to increase cardiac output and improve perfusion of vital organs. The strategy for clinical decision-making on the optimal treatment approach to increase cardiac output is based on pre-treatment blood pressure (Figure 10.1 and Table 10.1).

If the blood pressure is >120 mmHg (indicative of a very high systemic vascular resistance), then vasodilator therapy with intravenous nitroglycerin or nesir-itide is a reasonable first step. If hemodynamic data are available, the goal is to reduce the pulmonary capillary wedge pressure to 15–18 mmHg and increase the cardiac index to >2.5 l/min/m². Nitroglycerin typically requires titration to a range of 100–400 mcg/min to achieve these goals in patients with advanced heart failure.[10,11] Nitroprusside is also an effective vasodilator agent, but its clinical utility is limited by the potential for cyanide toxicity during prolonged infusion.[12] Nesiritide has a longer half-life than nitroglycerin and therefore requires a loading dose of 2 mcg/kg to achieve a rapid onset of action. The bolus can be skipped if a slower onset of action is acceptable. Nesiritide generally does not require upward titration from its starting dose of 0.01 mcg/kg/min, but it can be cautiously up-titrated in increments of 0.005 mcg/kg/min to a maximum dose of 0.03 mcg/kg/min if necessary.[13] The half-life of nesiritide is about 20 minutes, so evaluation of the full clinical response to up-titration or down-titration

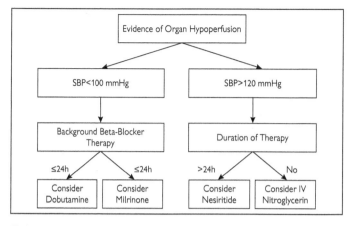

Figure 10.1 Schematic of therapeutic strategies for patients with advanced heart failure and low cardiac output syndrome. (See text for details.)

Table 10.1 Intravenous agents used to treat patients with low cardiac output syndrome

	Half-life (minutes)	Bolus Dose	Initial Infusion Dose	Maximum Infusion Dose
Vasodilator Agents				
Nitroglycerin	2–3	None	10 mcg/min	600 mcg/min
Nesiritide	18	2 mcg/kg	0.01 mcg/kg/min	0.03 mcg/kg/min
Positive Inotropic Agents				
Dobutamine	2	None	2.5 mcg/kg/min	15 mcg/kg/min
Milrinone	120	50 mcg/kg	0.5 mcg/kg/min*	0.75 mcg/kg/min
Positive Inotropic Agent with Renal Vasodilation				
Dopamine	2	None	2 mcg/kg/min	5 mcg/kg/min†

*Initial infusion dose is 0.375 mcg/kg/min in subjects with estimated glomerular filtration rate ≤30 ml/min and 0.25 mcg/kg/min in subjects with estimated glomerular filtration rate ≤20 ml/min.

†Higher doses may be used in the treatment of cardiogenic shock or other forms of shock. Above the dose of 5 mcg/kg/min, renal blood flow increases proportionately to the increase in cardiac output, so there is no selective renal perfusion effect.

of dose will require about two hours. If hemodynamic data are not available, clinical evidence of improved cardiac output includes patient symptoms (alleviation of restlessness and dyspnea), increased urine output, increased pulse pressure, increased pulse volume in the radial artery, resolution of pulsus alternans, increased warmth of the extremities, resolution of metabolic acidosis if present, and improved renal function. The major risk of vasodilator treatment is hypotension and consequent organ hypoperfusion/injury. The short half-life of nitroglycerin reduces risk of sustained hypotension. The longer half-life of nesiritide requires greater caution during initiation and up-titration, but survival was comparable to placebo in a large clinical trial of hospitalized patients with heart failure.[14]

If blood pressure is <100 mmHg (indicative of lower systemic vascular resistance), the agents with positive inotropic properties (dobutamine and milrinone) are useful to increase cardiac output. Dobutamine is a sympathomimetic agent that stimulates beta-1, beta-2, and alpha-1 adrenergic receptors.[15] Since the half-life of dobutamine is short, no bolus is required, and the drug can be rapidly titrated over its therapeutic range (2.5–15 mcg/kg/min). Dobutamine has a balanced effect on beta-2 and alpha-1 receptors in vascular smooth muscle, so it reduces systemic vascular resistance indirectly via baroreflex responses to increased cardiac output. Since dobutamine mediates its effects via adrenergic-receptor stimulation, its action will be attenuated in patients on beta-adrenergic-receptor blockers. Due to changes in the adrenergic receptor density and receptor coupling in failing myocardium, the response to dobutamine is heterogenous, and the dose must be individualized for each patient based on hemodynamic or clinical response. Dobutamine is generally well tolerated but can be associated with increased risk of arrhythmia and mild upper extremity tremor. Milrinone is a phosphodiesterase type 3 inhibitor that augments cyclic adenosine monophosphate signaling in myocardium and vascular smooth muscle.[16] The half-life of milrinone is approximately two hours, so a bolus of 50 mcg/kg (administered over 15–30 minutes) is required to achieve rapid action. The starting dose of milrinone is 0.5 mcg/kg/min (0.375 mcg/kg/min in patients with estimated glomerular filtration rate <30 ml/min). The dose can be titrated as necessary, but due to its long half-life, it will require nearly 12 hours to observe the full effect of the dose change. Accordingly, if a side effect of milrinone is suspected, it is appropriate to stop the infusion for two hours (one half-life) and resume at a lower dose. The half-life of milrinone is increased in patients with severely decreased renal function, so appropriate adjustments in dosing are necessary in that population. In contrast to dobutamine, milrinone has direct vasodilating activity in vascular smooth muscle, so it decreases systemic vascular resistance via both direct and indirect mechanisms. Since milrinone does not act by direct interaction with the beta-adrenergic receptor, its hemodynamic effects are preserved in patients treated with beta-adrenergic receptor antagonists.[17] Hemodynamic and clinical goals for both dobutamine and milrinone are the same as those described above for vasodilator agents. As dobutamine and milrinone mediate increased inotropy via the same final common pathway in the myocyte (increased cyclic adenosine monophosphate signaling), they share common side effects of positive chronotropy, and increased frequency of supraventricular and ventricular arrhythmias. Milrinone has additional potential side effects related to phosphodiesterase inhibition in the vasculature (hypotension) and gastrointestinal tract (nausea, vomiting, diarrhea). Both drugs can precipitate myocardial ischemia in patients with coronary artery disease, but the vasodilating action of milrinone decreases myocardial oxygen consumption compared with dobutamine.[18] Both dobutamine and milrinone have been associated with increased mortality risk in observational studies, so their use should be limited to patients with clear evidence of low cardiac output syndrome, with a strategy to use the lowest effective dose for the shortest possible time.

If the blood pressure is 100–120 mmHg, either vasodilator drugs or positive inotropic agents may be used, based on the estimated risk of symptomatic hypotension vs. potential adverse effects of positive inotropic agents.

Dopamine is an endogenous catecholamine with regional vasodilating action in the renal circulation. In patients with heart failure and low cardiac output syndrome, dopamine can be administered in low doses (1–3 mcg/kg/min) either alone or in combination with vasodilator agents or positive inotropic agents to increase renal perfusion and urine output.[19] Systemic side effects of low-dose dopamine are uncommon, but there is risk of severe local skin injury if there is extravasation of dopamine from a peripheral intravenous line. Ideally, dopamine should be infused via a central intravenous catheter, but if a peripheral venous catheter is used, the alpha-blocking agent phentolamine should be available for subcutaneous injection in case of extravasation to prevent intense vasoconstriction and ischemic skin injury. Other endogenous catecholamines including norepinephrine and epinephrine may be used in the setting of cardiogenic shock but are not routinely used in patients with low cardiac output syndrome.

The short-term goal for patients with low-cardiac-output syndrome is to utilize intravenous therapies to restore an optimal volume status, improve nutritional status and begin low-level exercise training to reverse deconditioning changes. In some patients, these goals can be achieved after three to five days of therapy, with transition back to an oral regimen at the time of hospital discharge. These patients remain at high risk for re-hospitalization, so preparation of advance directives and the possible need for referral for advanced surgical therapies (cardiac transplantation or mechanical circulatory support as discussed below) or referral to palliative care should be discussed. Some patients will manifest rapid return of the signs and symptoms of low-cardiac-output syndrome within hours to days after cessation of intravenous therapy, with resolution upon restarting of the intravenous therapy. These patients have a very high risk of death over the next year, so they should be considered for cardiac transplantation or mechanical circulatory support if eligible, or be considered for referral to palliative care in a hospice setting if not candidates for other advanced therapies. Intravenous therapies may be continued at home or at inpatient hospice settings as part of a comprehensive palliative care program (to include appropriate use of opiates for relief of pain, restlessness, and dyspnea). Continuous home infusion therapy may also be used in patients awaiting cardiac transplantation. Chronic venous access and collaboration with a visiting nursing service that can supply outpatient drug and home infusion pump is required. Intermittent outpatient infusions of positive inotropic agents or vasodilators have no proven benefit and are not recommended. For patients with implantable cardiovertor defibrillators, patients should be advised on the option of deactivating the device in the setting of end-stage disease.[20]

Heart transplantation is an effective intervention for patients with advanced heart failure refractory to other therapies.[21] A comprehensive evaluation to determine transplant eligibility is usually performed by the transplantation center. The major purpose of the evaluation is to confirm that the patient has end-stage disease refractory to all appropriate therapy and that the patient does not have another major disease or other life-limiting condition that would limit the likelihood of a successful transplantation procedure. Ongoing substance abuse (including tobacco), history of persistent non-adherence to medical therapy, poorly controlled major psychiatric illness, and other behavioral or psychosocial issues are relative contraindications to transplantation. Destination mechanical circulatory support with an implantable left-ventricular assist device is another option known to dramatically improve survival in patients with advanced heart failure.[22] A comprehensive evaluation similar to the transplantation evaluation is performed by the implant center. Eligibility guidelines differ for each center, but generally are somewhat less stringent than cardiac transplantation criteria and may include older patients (up to 80 years) and patients with moderate degrees of other organ dysfunction (for example, Stage 3–4 chronic kidney disease).

References

1. Perk G, Tunick PA, Kronzon I. Systolic and diastolic pulsus alternans in severe heart failure. *J Am Soc Echocardiogr.* 2007;20:905 e905–907.

2. Brack T, Thuer I, Clarenbach CF, et al. Daytime Cheyne-Stokes respiration in ambulatory patients with severe congestive heart failure is associated with increased mortality. *Chest.* 2007;132:1463–1471.

3. Aaronson KD, Schwartz JS, Chen TM, Wong KL, Goin JE, Mancini DM. Development and prospective validation of a clinical index to predict survival in ambulatory patients referred for cardiac transplant evaluation. *Circulation.* 1997;95:2660–2667.

4. Levy WC, Mozaffarian D, Linker DT, et al. The Seattle Heart Failure Model: prediction of survival in heart failure. *Circulation.* 2006;113:1424–1433.

5. Braunwald E. Biomarkers in heart failure. *N Engl J Med.* 2008;358:2148–2159.

6. Anker SD, Negassa A, Coats AJ, et al. Prognostic importance of weight loss in chronic heart failure and the effect of treatment with angiotensin-converting-enzyme inhibitors: an observational study. *Lancet.* 2003;361:1077–1083.

7. Horwich TB, Kalantar-Zadeh K, MacLellan RW, Fonarow GC. Albumin levels predict survival in patients with systolic heart failure. *Am Heart J.* 2008;155:883–889.

8. Tang YD, Katz SD. Anemia in chronic heart failure: prevalence, etiology, clinical correlates, and treatment options. *Circulation.* 2006;113:2454–2461.

9. Lewis GD, Murphy RM, Shah RV, et al. Pulmonary vascular response patterns during exercise in left-ventricular systolic dysfunction predict exercise capacity and outcomes. *Circ. Heart Fail.* 2011;4:276–285.

10. Packer M, Lee WH, Kessler PD, Gottlieb SS, Medina N, Yushak M. Prevention and reversal of nitrate tolerance in patients with congestive heart failure. *N Engl J Med.* 1987;317:799–804.

11. Intravenous nesiritide vs. nitroglycerin for treatment of decompensated congestive heart failure: a randomized controlled trial. *JAMA.* 2002;287:1531–1540.

12. Tinker JH, Michenfelder JD. Sodium nitroprusside: pharmacology, toxicology and therapeutics. *Anesthesiology.* 1976;45:340–354.

13. Colucci WS, Elkayam U, Horton DP, et al. Intravenous nesiritide, a natriuretic peptide, in the treatment of decompensated congestive heart failure. Nesiritide study group. *N Engl J Med.* 2000;343:246–253.

14. O'Connor CM, Starling RC, Hernandez AF, et al. Effect of nesiritide in patients with acute decompensated heart failure. *N Engl J Med.* 2011;365:32–43.

15. Sonnenblick EH, Frishman WH, LeJemtel TH. Dobutamine: a new synthetic cardioactive sympathetic amine. *N Engl J Med.* 1979;300:17–22.

16. Anderson JL, Baim DS, Fein SA, Goldstein RA, LeJemtel TH, Likoff MJ. Efficacy and safety of sustained (48-hour) intravenous infusions of milrinone in patients with severe congestive heart failure: a multicenter study. *J Am Coll Cardiol.* 1987;9:711–722.

17. Lowes BD, Tsvetkova T, Eichhorn EJ, Gilbert EM, Bristow MR. Milrinone versus dobutamine in heart failure subjects treated chronically with carvedilol. *Int J Cardiol.* 2001;81:141–149.

18. Grose R, Strain J, Greenberg M, LeJemtel TH. Systemic and coronary effects of intravenous milrinone and dobutamine in congestive heart failure. *J Am Coll Cardiol.* 1986;7:1107–1113.

19. Maskin CS, Ocken S, Chadwick B, LeJemtel TH. Comparative systemic and renal effects of dopamine and angiotensin-converting enzyme inhibition with enalaprilat in patients with heart failure. *Circulation.* 1985;72:846–852.

20. Lampert R, Hayes DL, Annas GJ, Farley MA, et al.; American Heart Association. HRS expert consensus statement on the management of cardiovascular implantable electronic devices (CIEDS) in patients nearing end of life or requesting withdrawal of therapy. *Heart Rhythm.* 2010;7:1008–1026.

21. Hunt SA. Taking heart—cardiac transplantation past, present, and future. *N Engl J Med.* 2006;355:231–235.

22. Fang JC. Rise of the machines—left-ventricular assist devices as permanent therapy for advanced heart failure. *N Engl J Med.* 2009;361:2282–2285.

Chapter 11

Management of Common Comorbidities in Patients with Chronic Heart Failure

Coronary Artery Disease

Coronary disease is the most common cause of heart failure with reduced ejection fraction, and is a common comorbid condition in patients with heart failure and preserved ejection fraction. The presence of comorbid coronary artery disease is associated with increased mortality risk, compared to heart failure patients without coronary artery disease.[1] Heart failure is a common complication of acute myocardial infarction. Loss of functioning myocytes during the acute myocardial infarction puts a greater load on the remaining myocytes remote from the infarction and initiates the process of ventricular remodeling with slowly progressive ventricular enlargement and decrease in left-ventricular ejection fraction over time.[2] Coronary artery disease may also impair diastolic relaxation and thus promote the progression of heart failure with preserved ejection fraction. The presence of heart failure during or after an acute myocardial infarction is associated with greater subsequent risk of heart failure and premature death.[1] Patients with acute myocardial infarction and evidence of left-ventricular systolic dysfunction (with or without clinical heart failure) should be treated with an angiotensin-converting enzyme inhibitor and beta-adrenergic-receptor blocking agent, as tolerated, during the index hospitalization and at discharge. A mineralocorticoid receptor antagonist should be added as tolerated to patients with symptomatic heart failure with reduced ejection fraction, or to asymptomatic patients with reduced ejection fraction and diabetes mellitus.[3] Patients should receive post-discharge treatment as described in chapters 7 through 9 for asymptomatic (Stage B) and symptomatic (Stage C) patients, respectively.

In patients with heart failure and symptomatic angina, it is reasonable to consider revascularization therapy with percutaneous intervention or surgical coronary-artery-bypass grafting as dictated by the coronary anatomy. Medical therapy for angina (in addition to beta-adrenergic-receptor blockers) may include various formulations of organic nitrates, and calcium blockers (amlodipine for low ejection fraction patients) as tolerated.[1] Ranolazine can be considered in patients with residual symptoms despite other anti-anginal therapy, or if low blood pressure limits the ability to titrate other classes of drugs.[4]

If the patient has obstructive coronary artery disease without symptomatic angina, the role of revascularization is less certain. Many heart failure patients with reduced ejection fraction and coronary artery disease have hypokinetic or akinetic segments of myocardium distal to coronary stenoses that may have the potential to increase contractile function if flow is restored with successful revascularization therapy ("hibernating myocardium"). Several imaging modalities have been developed to identify areas of viable myocardium whose contractile function may improve with revascularization (nuclear perfusion imaging, dobutamine stress echocardiography, PET assessment of myocardial glucose uptake, and cardiac MRI with contrast for assessment of full vs. partial thickness fibrosis and total scar burden), but there are limited head-to-head comparisons and no data from controlled prospective studies, so the optimal method or combination of methods has not been determined.[5] Interpretation of viability imaging should be considered in the context of the left-ventricular volumes, as there may be reduced benefit of revascularization in patients with more severe left-ventricular dilation.[6] The only prospective randomized trial of modern medical therapy vs. surgical revascularization therapy in patients with heart failure with reduced ejection fraction due to coronary artery disease did not demonstrate benefit with surgical therapy in patients with evidence of viable myocardium determined by radionuclide imaging or dobutamine stress echocardiography.[7] The findings of this trial (acronym STICH) remain controversial but are consistent with the findings of the earlier Occluded Artery Trial, in which the strategy of percutaneous intervention for occluded coronary arteries after myocardial infarction did not alter clinical outcomes when compared with optimal medical therapy in the subgroup of patients with post–myocardial infarction left-ventricular systolic dysfunction.[8] Accordingly, routine revascularization of heart failure patients without angina or angina-equivalent symptoms is not recommended. Decisions on revascularization in asymptomatic patients with heart failure with reduced ejection fraction and coronary artery disease must be made on an individual basis, with recognition of the limitations of the currently available imaging techniques for determining myocardial viability.

Aspirin is recommended as secondary prevention therapy after myocardial infarction. In patients with heart failure and reduced ejection fraction, there is concern that cyclooxygenase-inhibition with aspirin may attenuate benefits of angiotensin-converting enzyme inhibitors.[9,10] There are no prospective randomized studies in the heart failure population, and evidence from retrospective analyses regarding the benefits and risks of aspirin in this population is inconsistent. It is recommended to continue low-dose aspirin (81 mg daily) in patients with heart failure and known coronary artery disease. Thienopyridines should be used according to indications related to recent myocardial infarction or history of coronary stent placement, as there is no other proven role either alone or in addition to aspirin in the chronic heart failure population. Warfarin therapy is reasonable to consider for patients with atrial fibrillation or history of thromboembolic events, but it was not superior to aspirin for reduction in mortality in patients with chronic heart failure with reduced ejection fraction in sinus rhythm.[11,12]

The role of lipid-lowering therapy with HMG-CoA reductase inhibitors (statins) in patients with heart failure is controversial, as two large, randomized clinical trials demonstrated that treatment with a high-potency statin (rosuvastatin) failed to improve cardiac outcomes over placebo in patients with heart failure and low ejection fraction.[13,14] There are no comparable prospective clinical trial data for patients with heart failure and preserved ejection fraction, but observational studies suggest the potential benefit of statins in this population.[15] Accordingly, decision on lipid-lowering therapy with statins in patients with heart failure should be individualized based on assessment of the long-term prognosis, left-ventricular ejection fraction, and estimated risk of recurrent ischemic events. N-3 polyunsaturated fatty acid (fish oil) supplements may also be considered in the heart failure populations. Studies in patients with heart failure and reduced ejection fraction have demonstrated short-term benefit on function class and possibly small reductions in adverse clinical outcome events with n-3 polyunsaturated fatty acid supplements when compared with placebo.[16] Additional clinical trials are needed to determine whether n-3 polyunsaturated fatty acid supplements should be routinely administered to all patients with heart failure and reduced ejection fraction.

Hypertension

Hypertension is the most common risk factor for development of heart failure and is a common comorbidity in patients with heart failure with preserved ejection fraction.[17] In the hypertension population, left-ventricular hypertrophy detected by electrocardiography or echocardiography is associated with increased risk of incident heart failure.

Treatment of hypertension has been shown to reduce the risk of developing heart failure. A network meta-analysis of over 200,000 subjects in randomized clinical trials indicates that the risk of heart failure is reduced with all classes of drugs except alpha-blockers, with greatest reduction of risk associated with thiazide diuretics and angiotensin-converting enzyme inhibitors or angiotensin-receptor blockers.[18]

In patients with chronic heart failure, more stringent goals for blood pressure lowering are recommended (goal: <130/80). For hypertensive patients with reduced ejection fraction, there are compelling indications to use the combination of beta-adrenergic-receptor blockers with either angiotensin-converting enzyme inhibitors or angiotensin-receptor blockers as first-line agents for blood pressure control, based on the results of outcomes studies reviewed in chapters 7, 8, and 9. For hypertensive patients with preserved ejection fraction, it is reasonable to consider use of beta-adrenergic-receptor blockers and either angiotensin-converting enzyme inhibitor or angiotensin-receptor blocker therapy, but there are no prospective data demonstrating differential survival benefits for these classes of agents. Diuretics including thiazide diuretics should also be considered in patients with preserved ejection fraction and history of volume overload. For the subgroup of hypertensive patients with left-ventricular hypertrophy (but not symptomatic heart failure, Stage B), losartan therapy (plus thiazide diuretic and other agents as needed) was associated with greater reduction in left-ventricular hypertrophy (determined by electrocardiographic or echocardiographic criteria); it was also associated with a reduced risk of death or nonfatal heart attack or stroke when compared with atenolol therapy (plus thiazide diuretic and other agents as needed), despite comparable reductions in blood pressure. These findings support preferential use of an angiotensin-receptor blocker as first-line agent in this subgroup.

Valvular Heart Disease

Mitral regurgitation due to dilation of the mitral valve annulus is a common comorbidity in patients with heart failure and reduced ejection fraction and is associated with increased mortality risk.[19] A large regurgitant volume associated with severe mitral regurgitation may be associated with increased left-ventricular remodeling and disease progression. Therapeutic strategies are based on the presence of symptoms, the severity of the regurgitation (size of the regurgitant volume), valve anatomy, and the assessment of ventricular size and function.

In many patients, the severity of mitral regurgitation is dynamic, with increased regurgitation fraction in response to increased preload and/or afterload.[20] Accordingly, the severity of mitral regurgitation should be assessed on optimal medical therapy. Echocardiography (transthoracic and/or transesophageal), contrast ventriculography, and cardiac MRI may be used to assess the severity of mitral regurgitation. Each imaging technique has strengths and weaknesses, and an integrated multimodality approach is recommended for most patients.[21,22]

Current guidelines recommend mitral valve surgery (replacement or repair) for symptomatic patients with severe mitral regurgitation and left-ventricular ejection fraction ≥30% and/or end-systolic left-ventricular dimension ≤55 mm. For patients with mitral regurgitation and more severe left-ventricular systolic dysfunction, there is no evidence that mitral valve surgery is associated with improved survival.[23] Percutaneous mitral valve clip procedures have been evaluated for patients who meet standard surgical criteria, but not for patients with more severe left-ventricular systolic function.[24]

Atrial Fibrillation

Atrial fibrillation is present in nearly one-third of patients with heart failure and is associated with increased mortality risk.[25] Atrial fibrillation in heart failure patients is associated with greater stroke risk than in patients without heart failure and in heart failure patients in sinus rhythm. Accordingly, chronic oral anticoagulation therapy is recommended for this population unless there is a specific contraindication or intolerance. For patients unable to tolerate oral anticoagulation, alternative therapies, including aspirin, implantation of left-atrial-appendage occlusion device, or surgical ligation of the left atrial appendage, can be considered.[26] For patients with a new diagnosis of atrial fibrillation (paroxysmal, persistent, or permanent), it is important to evaluate them for potentially correctable exacerbating factors (thyroid disease, worsening valvular heart disease, pericardial disease, pulmonary embolism, obstructive sleep apnea, acute and/or chronic alcohol abuse, other substance abuse).[27]

For most patients with atrial fibrillation, chronic heart failure with low ejection fraction, and stable symptoms, rate control with medical therapy is a reasonable initial strategy.[28] The optimal target heart rate for the rate control strategy has not been determined, but a goal of less than 80 beats per minute at rest, and under 110 beats per minute during moderate exercise, is reasonable and attainable in most patients.[29,30] A regimen of a beta-adrenergic-receptor blockade and digoxin, medications indicated for the underlying diagnosis of low ejection fraction heart failure, is often an effective rate control regimen. In an emergent setting, cautious dosing of intravenous diltiazem or intravenous amiodarone can also be considered. Amiodarone can also be considered for chronic rate control, although its use is considered second-line due to the known toxicities associated with long-term amiodarone use.[31] Diltiazem and verapamil are often poorly tolerated for chronic rate control in patients with reduced ejection fraction. In rare instances where drug therapy is either ineffective or not tolerated, atrioventricular node ablation with implantation of a permanent electronic pacemaker can be considered for rate control.

If effective rate control cannot be achieved, or if atrial fibrillation with controlled rate is associated with decreased functional capacity or symptomatic palpitations, it is reasonable to consider rhythm control strategies to reduce symptoms. Electrical cardioversion in conjunction with transesophageal echocardiography for imaging the left atrial appendage thrombus is the preferred technique for restoring sinus rhythm. Amiodarone is an effective antiarrhythmic agent for conversion to and maintenance of sinus rhythm and has a good safety record in heart failure. Amiodarone requires a loading dose (600 mg–800 mg daily for total dose of 10 gm), which can be administered to an outpatient with careful monitoring of the QT interval.[31] Digoxin dose should be halved at the time of initiation of amiodarone therapy, with careful monitoring of digoxin serum levels. Coumadin dosing must also be carefully monitored at the time of initiation of amiodarone therapy. Dofetilide has also been shown to be an effective rhythm control agent for atrial fibrillation in heart failure. Due to risks of prorhythmia (3%–4% in a placebo-controlled trial), dofetilide therapy should be initiated in an inpatient setting with telemetry monitoring and dose adjustment according to QT interval and renal function.[32,33] Catheter-based ablation of atrial fibrillation or related atrial ablation surgical procedures performed at the time of open heart surgery are effective alternative therapies for rhythm control, although the long-term effects of this approach on clinical outcomes have not yet been determined.[34]

Management of patients with atrial fibrillation, heart failure and preserved ejection fraction, and stable symptoms, is for the most part comparable to management of patients with reduced ejection fraction. In the setting of preserved ejection fraction, non-dihydropyridine calcium channel blockers (diltiazem, verapamil) may be used for chronic rate control as alternatives to, or in combination with, beta-adrenergic blockers. Digoxin may also be considered for rate control in this group. There are limited data on the safety of available rhythm control agents in this population. In addition to amiodarone, other agents, including sotalol, dofetilide, propafenone, and flecainide, may be considered, based on the presence of structural heart disease and coronary artery disease.[29,30]

Ventricular Arrhythmias

Complex ventricular ectopy, including non-sustained ventricular tachycardia, is nearly ubiquitous in patients with heart failure and reduced ejection fraction and therefore does not have strong predictive value for risk of sudden death apart from that conferred by the degree of left-ventricular systolic dysfunction.[35] Implantable defibrillators are recommended as primary prevention for symptomatic patients with left-ventricular ejection fraction <35%, regardless of the presence or absence of ventricular ectopy.[36] In patients with a history of frequent firing of the implantable cardiovertor defibrillator, anti-arrhythmic therapy with anti-arrhythmic agents or ablation should be considered. Device therapy is not recommended for patients with heart failure and preserved ejection fraction, except in the case of a sudden-death survivor.

Very frequent ectopic beats may be associated with impaired ventricular function and worsened functional capacity, presumably related to atrio-ventricular dyssynchrony and ventriculo-ventricular dyssynchrony of the ectopic beats.[37] If the majority of the ectopic beats are monomorphic, ablation of the ventricular focus of the ectopy may be associated with improved ventricular function and improved functional capacity.[38] Frequent monomorphic ventricular beats arising from the right-ventricular outflow tract may confer risk of worsening systolic dysfunction and symptomatic events, so referral to an electrophysiologist for further evaluation and possible ablation therapy is recommended.[39]

Chronic Kidney Disease

Chronic kidney disease is a common comorbid condition in patients with heart failure and is associated with increased mortality risk, with greater risk in the patients with preserved ejection fraction.[40,41] The pathogenesis of chronic kidney disease in the heart failure patient is complex. Hypertension and diabetes mellitus are common risk factors for both heart and kidney disease. Altered hemodynamics and neurohormonal activation in heart failure may exacerbate progression of kidney disease. Increased salt and water retention in chronic kidney disease can exacerbate congestive symptoms and also promote disease progression.

Chronic kidney disease is often associated with diuretic resistance that complicates management. The pathophysiology of diuretic resistance is probably multifactorial and attributable to decreased nephron mass with reduced amount of filtered sodium, abnormal intraglomerular hemodynamics, neurohormonal activation, and abnormal central hemodynamics that reduce renal blood flow. Treatment of volume overload often requires very high doses of loop diuretics and/or combination therapy of a loop diuretic with a thiazide diuretic. Serum creatinine levels often increase in response to effective diuretic therapy in this population. The rise in creatinine may be related to intrarenal effects of furosemide (tubuloglomerular feedback), hemodynamic effects related to decongestion (reduced cardiac output in response to preload reduction), and/or creatinine concentration effects related to reduction in total body water during a large-volume diuresis. Importantly, none of these mechanisms are associated with permanent renal injury. Indeed, experimental studies consistently demonstrate that loop diuretics protect the kidney from ischemic tubular injury. Accordingly, diuretics should be titrated to relief of congestive signs and symptoms, even in the face of rising creatinine, if there is no other evidence of oliguria or acute kidney injury. Ultrafiltration can be considered as an alternative to diuretic therapy, but this should be implemented in consultation with a nephrologist in this population. Repeated central venous access or PICC-line placement for ultrafiltration may cause central venous thrombosis that could complicate vascular access for future hemodialysis in the event of progression to end-stage kidney disease. Available evidence suggests that the risk of worsening renal function during decongestion with loop diuretics and ultrafiltration are comparable.

Chronic kidney disease may also impact the use of pharmacological inhibitors of the renin-angiotensin-aldosterone axis in patients with heart failure.[42] There are limited data on the effects of angiotensin converting enzyme (ACE) inhibitors in patients with heart failure and chronic kidney disease, as most clinical trials excluded patients with serum creatinine >2.5 mg/dl. The ACE inhibitor benazepril was demonstrated to slow progression of renal disease in chronic kidney disease patients with starting serum creatinine between 3.1–5.0 mg/dl.[43] Observational studies suggest that ACE inhibition (or angiotensin receptor blocker (ARB) therapy) is associated with decreased mortality risk in patients with chronic systolic heart failure and chronic kidney disease, including patients with more severe chronic kidney disease.[44,45] Accordingly, ACE inhibition (or ARB therapy) is recommended in this population, with recognition that a small initial decrease in estimated glomerular filtration rate is expected, and that careful long-term monitoring of renal function and serum potassium levels is required. Potassium supplement doses should be reduced or discontinued. Patients should receive instructions for a low-sodium, low-potassium diet and should not use salt substitutes that contain potassium chloride. Mineralocorticoid receptor antagonists are also associated with an increased risk of worsening renal function and hyperkalemia in patients with chronic kidney disease, but they may be used with caution in combination with ACE inhibitors (or ARB therapy) in patients with estimated creatinine clearance 30–60 ml/min.

Anemia

Prevalence of anemia increases in proportion to the severity of heart failure symptoms.[46] The etiology of anemia is dilutional in about half the cases, and related to chronic disease (including chronic kidney disease) and iron deficiency in another 25%–35%. Angiotensin-converting-enzyme inhibitors are also known to suppress red blood cell production and are therefore likely contribute to the anemia. Anemia has been identified as an independent predictor of increased mortality risk in the heart failure population.[47]

Treatment of anemia should be directed at the underlying cause. In patients with hemodilution, increased diuretic therapy to achieve optimal volume status may be sufficient treatment. Small studies indicate that erythropoietic stimulating agents (ESAs) can increase hemoglobin and improve exercise tolerance in patients with heart failure, but correction of anemia with long-term ESA therapy does not improve survival when compared with placebo in patients with heart failure and reduced ejection fraction.[48] In patients with concomitant chronic kidney disease, erythropoietic stimulating agents can be used in accordance with existing guidelines for that population with target hemoglobin of 10–11 mg/dl.[49] If iron deficiency is identified, intravenous iron preparations, rather than oral iron preparations, should be used to replenish iron stores, since oral iron is very poorly absorbed in patients with heart failure.[50] Iron dextran has a small but non-negligible risk of life-threatening anaphylaxis, so it should no longer be used. Other forms of intravenous iron, including iron sucrose and iron gluconate, are well tolerated and can be administered on an outpatient basis to replenish iron stores. Intravenous iron supplementation has also been shown to be associated with improved functional capacity in patients with functional iron deficiency and normal hemoglobin levels. However, the long-term safety of this approach has not yet been determined, so it is not recommended for clinical practice at this time.

Diabetes Mellitus

Diabetes mellitus is present in 20%–40% of patients with heart failure and is associated with increased mortality risk in patients with heart failure with both preserved and reduced ejection fraction.[51,52] Diabetes mellitus may contribute to heart failure progression through direct effects on myocardial metabolism, substrate utilization, and mitochondrial energetics, and/or indirectly through its promotion of atherosclerosis progression and chronic kidney disease.

Better glycemic control, as assessed by hemoglobin A_{1c} levels, is associated with improved clinical outcomes in patients with heart failure and diabetes mellitus.[52,53] However, there are limited data to guide therapeutic choices for management of diabetes in the heart failure population.[54] Sulfonylureas are generally well tolerated and appear to be safe for the heart failure population. Metformin carries an FDA warning about use in heart failure patients due to concern over the risk of development of lactic acidosis. However, post-marketing surveillance revealed a very low risk of lactic acidosis in clinical practice (5 cases per 100,000 treated patients), and observational studies suggest that metformin use is associated with reduced mortality risk in diabetic heart failure patients.[55] Thiazolidinediones (TZDs) are associated with edema formation and are not recommended for use in patients with heart failure.[54] A meta-analysis of randomized clinical trials demonstrated that TZD use in diabetics is associated with increased risk of clinical heart failure, but not cardiovascular mortality. Observational studies suggest that TZD use is not associated with increased mortality risk in heart failure populations. Until additional prospective data become available, it is reasonable to consider TZD use in selected patients with less severe symptoms, with close follow-up of volume status and adjustment in diuretic dose as needed. The role of insulin therapy in diabetic heart failure patients is uncertain, as existing reports have yielded conflicting data with regard to the association between insulin use and mortality risk.[54]

Chronic Obstructive Lung Disease

Chronic obstructive lung disease is a common comorbidity in patients with chronic heart failure with both preserved and reduced ejection fraction.[56–58] Estimates of the prevalence of chronic obstructive lung disease in heart failure range from 20%–40%, but the accuracy of this estimate remains uncertain due to the diagnostic challenges discussed below. The presence of comorbid chronic obstructive lung disease is associated with increased mortality risk in patients with heart failure.

Dyspnea and exercise intolerance are common symptoms associated with both chronic lung disease and heart failure.[56–58] In chronic lung disease, abnormal gas exchange at rest or during exercise leads to arterial oxygen desaturation and reduced oxygen delivery to active skeletal muscle. In chronic heart disease, arterial oxygen desaturation does not occur during exercise, but oxygen delivery to active skeletal muscle is limited by reduced cardiac output reserve. In both disease states, low-grade inflammation, cachexia, and skeletal muscle atrophy also contribute to exercise intolerance. Clinical determination of the cause of dyspnea in patients with both chronic lung and heart disease is difficult due to overlapping symptoms and the non-specific findings on physical examination. Accordingly, one must maintain a high level of suspicion for detection of comorbid disease in both populations. For patients with lung disease, measurement of brain natriuretic peptide can be clinically useful, as very high (>500 pg/ml) or very low values (<100 pg/ml) can alter the post-test probability of comorbid heart disease. Measurement of left-ventricular ejection fraction with echocardiography (or, if acoustic windows are limited by emphysematous lung disease, with radionuclide ventriculography or cardiac MRI) should be considered, as identification of reduced ejection fraction would change the therapeutic strategy. As discussed in previous chapters, the presence of a preserved ejection fraction does not rule out heart failure. If the diagnosis remains in doubt despite biomarkers and cardiac imaging, exercise testing with analysis of expired gases and arterial oxygen saturation, and/or right-heart catheterization can be considered.

The presence of lung disease (chronic obstructive lung disease and/or asthma) is often cited as a contraindication to the use of beta-adrenergic-receptor antagonists.[56–58] There are limited data available on the use of beta-adrenergic blockers in patients with heart failure and chronic lung disease; however, the bulk of available evidence suggests that cardioselective beta-1 adrenergic blockers can be used safely in this population, even in patients with evidence of reversible air flow obstruction in response to beta-2 agonists. The available data support the preferential use of long-acting metoprolol succinate or bisoprolol over carvedilol in this population.[59,60]

Cough is a common symptom in patients with chronic lung disease; it is also common in patients with chronic heart failure, and is among the most common complications of ACE inhibition therapy (estimated to occur in 10%–20% of treated patients). Accordingly, a careful history must be taken to distinguish the cause of cough in a patient with heart failure and comorbid lung disease. The cough associated with ACE inhibition is typically non-productive and can be provoked by speaking, ingestion of cold liquids, or inhalation of cold air. Most important, the cough associated with ACE inhibition will rapidly dissipate after discontinuation of therapy. Limited data from small prospective studies and post-marking registries suggest that the risk of cough (or, more rarely, bronchospasm) associated with ACE inhibition is not increased in patients with heart failure and comorbid chronic lung disease. If the etiology of a persistent cough remains uncertain, an angiotensin-receptor antagonist can be substituted.[61]

Sleep-Disordered Breathing

Sleep-disordered breathing (obstructive and/or central sleep apnea) is a common comorbid condition in patients with heart failure with both preserved and reduced ejection fraction, and is associated with increased mortality risk.[62–64] Recurrent hypoxic events during sleep can exacerbate daytime fatigue, increase blood pressure, increase pulmonary artery pressure, and promote sodium retention and volume overload.

Both central and obstructive sleep apnea are common, so a sleep study is indicated to determine the severity and type(s) of sleep apnea present. Patients with complaints of daytime somnolence, obesity, difficult-to-control hypertension, diuretic resistance, and pulmonary hypertension should be considered for evaluation in a sleep laboratory. Absence of daytime somnolence is not by itself sufficient to exclude the presence of nocturnal apnea.[65]

Positive airway pressure (PAP) breathing has been shown to improve symptoms in patients with heart failure and reduced ejection fraction, but was not associated with improved survival.[66] Adherence to positive pressure breathing masks in clinical practice can be limited by patient intolerance.

References

1. Gheorghiade M, Sopko G, De Luca L, et al. Navigating the crossroads of coronary artery disease and heart failure. *Circulation.* 2006;114:1202–1213.

2. Pfeffer MA. Left-ventricular remodeling after acute myocardial infarction. *Ann Rev Med.* 1995;46:455–466.

3. Pitt B, Remme W, Zannad F, Neaton J, et al. Eplerenone, a selective aldosterone blocker, in patients with left-ventricular dysfunction after myocardial infarction. *N Engl J Med.* 2003;348:1309–1321.

4. Keating GM. Ranolazine: a review of its use in chronic stable angina pectoris. *Drugs.* 2008;68:2483–2503.

5. Rahimtoola SH, Dilsizian V, Kramer CM, Marwick TH, Vanoverschelde JL. Chronic ischemic left-ventricular dysfunction: from pathophysiology to imaging and its integration into clinical practice. *J Am Coll Cardiol. Cardiovasc Imaging.* 2008;1:536–555.

6. Kwon DH, Hachamovitch R, Popovic ZB, et al. Survival in patients with severe ischemic cardiomyopathy undergoing revascularization versus medical therapy: association with end-systolic volume and viability. *Circulation.* 2012;126:S3–S8.

7. Bonow RO, Maurer G, Lee KL, et al. Myocardial viability and survival in ischemic left-ventricular dysfunction. *N Engl J Med.* 2011;364:1617–1625.

8. Kruk M, Buller CE, Tcheng JE, et al. Impact of left-ventricular ejection fraction on clinical outcomes over five years after infarct-related coronary

artery recanalization (from the Occluded Artery Trial [OAT]). *Am J Cardiol.* 2010;105:10–16.

9. Massie BM. Aspirin use in chronic heart failure: what should we recommend to the practitioner? *J Am Coll Cardiol.* 2005;46:963–966.

10. Stys T, Lawson WE, Smaldone GC, Stys A. Does aspirin attenuate the beneficial effects of angiotensin-converting enzyme inhibition in heart failure? *Arch Intern Med.* 2000;160:1409–1413.

11. Homma S, Thompson JL, Pullicino PM, et al. Warfarin and aspirin in patients with heart failure and sinus rhythm. *N Engl J Med.* 2012;366:1859–1869.

12. Massie BM, Collins JF, Ammon SE, et al. Randomized trial of warfarin, aspirin, and clopidogrel in patients with chronic heart failure: the Warfarin and Antiplatelet Therapy in Chronic Heart Failure (WATCH) trial. *Circulation.* 2009;119:1616–1624.

13. Kjekshus J, Apetrei E, Barrios V, et al. Rosuvastatin in older patients with systolic heart failure. *N Engl J Med.* 2007;357:2248–2261.

14. Tavazzi L, Maggioni AP, Marchioli R, et al. Effect of rosuvastatin in patients with chronic heart failure (the GISSI-HF trial): A randomised, double-blind, placebo-controlled trial. *Lancet.* 2008;372:1231–1239.

15. Tehrani F, Morrissey R, Phan A, Chien C, Schwarz ER. Statin therapy in patients with diastolic heart failure. *Clin Cardiol.* 2010;33:E1–E5.

16. Tavazzi L, Maggioni AP, Marchioli R, et al. Effect of n-3 polyunsaturated fatty acids in patients with chronic heart failure (the GISSI-HF trial): A randomised, double-blind, placebo-controlled trial. *Lancet.* 2008;372:1223–1230.

17. Klapholz M, Maurer M, Lowe AM, et al. Hospitalization for heart failure in the presence of a normal left ventricular ejection fraction: results of the New York Heart Failure Registry. *J Am Coll Cardiol.* 2004;43:1432–1438.

18. Sciarretta S, Palano F, Tocci G, Baldini R, Volpe M. Antihypertensive treatment and development of heart failure in hypertension: A Bayesian network meta-analysis of studies in patients with hypertension and high cardiovascular risk. *Arch Intern Med.* 2011;171:384–394.

19. Trichon BH, Felker GM, Shaw LK, Cabell CH, O'Connor CM. Relation of frequency and severity of mitral regurgitation to survival among patients with left-ventricular systolic dysfunction and heart failure. *Am J Cardiol.* 2003;91:538–543.

20. Keren G, Katz S, Strom J, Sonnenblick EH, LeJemtel TH. Dynamic mitral regurgitation. An important determinant of the hemodynamic response to load alterations and inotropic therapy in severe heart failure. *Circulation.* 1989;80:306–313.

21. Apostolakis EE, Baikoussis NG. Methods of estimation of mitral valve regurgitation for the cardiac surgeon. *J Cardiothorac Surg.* 2009;4:34.

22. Grayburn PA, Weissman NJ, Zamorano JL. Quantitation of mitral regurgitation. *Circulation.* 2012;126:2005–2017.

23. Wu AH, Aaronson KD, Bolling SF, Pagani FD, Welch K, Koelling TM. Impact of mitral valve annuloplasty on mortality risk in patients with mitral regurgitation and left-ventricular systolic dysfunction. *J Am Coll Cardiol.* 2005;45:381–387.

24. Feldman T, Foster E, Glower DD, et al. Percutaneous repair or surgery for mitral regurgitation. *N Engl J Med.* 2011;364:1395–1406.

25. Camm AJ, Savelieva I, Lip GY. Rate control in the medical management of atrial fibrillation. *Heart.* 2007;93:35–38.

26. Aryana A, Saad EB, d'Avila A. Left atrial appendage occlusion and ligation devices: what is available, how to implement them, and how to manage and avoid complications. *Curr Treat Options Cardiovasc Med.* 2012;14:503–519.

27. Callahan T, Baranowski B. Managing newly diagnosed atrial fibrillation: rate, rhythm, and risk. *Cleve Clin J Med.* 2011;78:258–264.

28. Roy D, Talajic M, Nattel S, et al. Rhythm control versus rate control for atrial fibrillation and heart failure. *N Engl J Med.* 2008;358:2667–2677.

29. Fuster V, Ryden LE, Cannom DS, et al. 2011 ACCF/AHA/HRS focused updates incorporated into the ACC/AHA/ESC 2006 guidelines for the management of patients with atrial fibrillation: a report of the American College of Cardiology Foundation/American Heart Association task force on practice guidelines. *Circulation.* 2011;123:e269–e367.

30. Fuster V, Ryden LE, Cannom DS, et al. ACC/AHA/ESC 2006 guidelines for the management of patients with atrial fibrillation: a report of the American College of Cardiology/American Heart Association task force on practice guidelines and the European Society of Cardiology Committee for Practice Guidelines (writing committee to revise the 2001 guidelines for the management of patients with atrial fibrillation): developed in collaboration with the European Heart Rhythm Association and the Heart Rhythm Society. *Circulation.* 2006;114:e257–e354.

31. Siddoway LA. Amiodarone: Guidelines for use and monitoring. *Am Fam Physician.* 2003;68:2189–2196.

32. Grines CL. Safety and effectiveness of dofetilide for conversion of atrial fibrillation and nesiritide for acute decompensation of heart failure: a report from the Cardiovascular and Renal Advisory Panel of the Food and Drug Administration. *Circulation.* 2000;101:E200–E201.

33. Torp-Pedersen C, Moller M, Bloch-Thomsen PE, et al. Dofetilide in patients with congestive heart failure and left-ventricular dysfunction. Danish Investigations of Arrhythmia and Mortality on Dofetilide study group. *N Engl J Med.* 1999;341:857–865.

34. Chinitz JS, Halperin JL, Reddy VY, Fuster V. Rate or rhythm control for atrial fibrillation: Update and controversies. *Am J Med.* November, 2012;125(11):1049–1056.

35. Olshausen KV, Stienen U, Schwarz F, Kubler W, Meyer J. Long-term prognostic significance of ventricular arrhythmias in idiopathic dilated cardiomyopathy. *Am J Cardiol.* 1988;61:146–151.

36. Bardy GH, Lee KL, Mark DB, et al. Amiodarone or an implantable cardioverter-defibrillator for congestive heart failure. *N Engl J Med.* 2005;352:225–237.

37. Baman TS, Lange DC, Ilg KJ, et al. Relationship between burden of premature ventricular complexes and left-ventricular function. *Heart Rhythm.* 2010;7:865–869.

38. Wijnmaalen AP, Delgado V, Schalij MJ, et al. Beneficial effects of catheter ablation on left-ventricular and right ventricular function in patients with frequent premature ventricular contractions and preserved ejection fraction. *Heart.* 2010;96:1275–1280.

39. Yarlagadda RK, Iwai S, Stein KM, et al. Reversal of cardiomyopathy in patients with repetitive monomorphic ventricular ectopy originating from the right ventricular outflow tract. *Circulation.* 2005;112:1092–1097.

40. Ahmed A, Rich MW, Sanders PW, et al. Chronic kidney disease associated mortality in diastolic versus systolic heart failure: a propensity matched study. *Am J Cardiol.* 2007;99:393–398.

41. Herzog CA, Muster HA, Li S, Collins AJ. Impact of congestive heart failure, chronic kidney disease, and anemia on survival in the Medicare population. *J Card Fail.* 2004;10:467–472.

42. Abdo AS, Basu A, Geraci SA. Managing chronic heart failure patient in chronic kidney disease. *Am J Med.* 2011;124:26–28.

43. Hou FF, Zhang X, Zhang GH, et al. Efficacy and safety of benazepril for advanced chronic renal insufficiency. *N Engl J Med.* 2006;354:131–140.

44. Ahmed A, Fonarow GC, Zhang Y, et al. Renin-angiotensin inhibition in systolic heart failure and chronic kidney disease. *Am J Med.* 2012;125:399–410.

45. Ahmed A, Love TE, Sui X, Rich MW. Effects of angiotensin-converting enzyme inhibitors in systolic heart failure patients with chronic kidney disease: a propensity score analysis. *Journal of cardiac failure.* 2006;12:499–506.

46. Tang YD, Katz SD. Anemia in chronic heart failure: prevalence, etiology, clinical correlates, and treatment options. *Circulation.* 2006;113:2454–2461.

47. Anand I, McMurray JJ, Whitmore J, et al. Anemia and its relationship to clinical outcome in heart failure. *Circulation.* 2004;110:149–154.

48. Swedberg K, Young JB, Anand IS, et al. Treatment of anemia with darbepoetin alfa in systolic heart failure. *N Engl J Med* 2013, ePub before print.

49. Kidney Disease Outcomes Quality Initiative (KDOQI) clinical practice guidelines and clinical practice recommendations for anemia in chronic kidney disease. *Am J Kidney Dis.* 2006;47:S11–S145.

50. Jelani QU, Attanasio P, Katz SD, Anker SD. Treatment with iron of patients with heart failure with and without anemia. *Heart Fail Clin.* 2010;6:305–312.

51. MacDonald MR, Petrie MC, Varyani F, et al. Impact of diabetes on outcomes in patients with low and preserved ejection fraction heart failure: an analysis of the Candesartan in Heart Failure: Assessment of Reduction in Mortality and Morbidity (CHARM) programme. *Eur Heart J.* 2008;29:1377–1385.

52. Romero SP, Garcia-Egido A, Escobar MA, et al. Impact of new-onset diabetes mellitus and glycemic control on the prognosis of heart failure patients: a propensity-matched study in the community. *Int J Cardiol.* 2012.

53. Tomova GS, Nimbal V, Horwich TB. Relation between hemoglobin A1C and outcomes in heart failure patients with and without diabetes mellitus. *Am J Cardiol.* 2012;109:1767–1773.

54. MacDonald MR, Petrie MC, Hawkins NM, et al. Diabetes, left-ventricular systolic dysfunction, and chronic heart failure. *Eur Heart J.* 2008;29:1224–1240.

55. Aguilar D, Chan W, Bozkurt B, Ramasubbu K, Deswal A. Metformin use and mortality in ambulatory patients with diabetes and heart failure. *Circ. Heart Fail.* 2011;4:53–58.

56. Hawkins NM, Petrie MC, Macdonald MR, et al. Heart failure and chronic obstructive pulmonary disease the quandary of beta-blockers and beta-agonists. *J Am Coll Cardiol.* 2011;57:2127–2138.

57. Le Jemtel TH, Padeletti M, Jelic S. Diagnostic and therapeutic challenges in patients with coexistent chronic obstructive pulmonary disease and chronic heart failure. *J Am Coll Cardiol.* 2007;49:171–180.

58. Mascarenhas J, Azevedo A, Bettencourt P. Coexisting chronic obstructive pulmonary disease and heart failure: Implications for treatment, course and mortality. *Curr Opin Pulm Med.* 2010;16:106–111.

59. Hawkins NM, MacDonald MR, Petrie MC, et al. Bisoprolol in patients with heart failure and moderate to severe chronic obstructive pulmonary disease: a randomized controlled trial. *Eur J Heart Fail.* 2009;11:684–690.

60. Kotlyar E, Keogh AM, Macdonald PS, Arnold RH, McCaffrey DJ, Glanville AR. Tolerability of carvedilol in patients with heart failure and concomitant chronic obstructive pulmonary disease or asthma. *J Heart Lung Transplant.* 2002;21:1290–1295.

61. Packard KA, Wurdeman RL, Arouni AJ. ACE inhibitor–induced bronchial reactivity in patients with respiratory dysfunction. *Ann Pharmacother.* 2002;36:1058–1067.

62. Herrscher TE, Akre H, Overland B, Sandvik L, Westheim AS. High prevalence of sleep apnea in heart failure outpatients: even in patients with preserved systolic function. *J Card Fail.* 2011;17:420–425.

63. McKelvie RS, Moe GW, Cheung A, et al. The 2011 Canadian Cardiovascular Society heart failure management guidelines update: focus on sleep apnea, renal dysfunction, mechanical circulatory support, and palliative care. *Can J Cardiol.* 2011;27:319–338.

64. Wang H, Parker JD, Newton GE, et al. Influence of obstructive sleep apnea on mortality in patients with heart failure. *J Am Coll Cardiol.* 2007;49:1625–1631.

65. Arzt M, Young T, Finn L, et al. Sleepiness and sleep in patients with both systolic heart failure and obstructive sleep apnea. *Arch Intern Med.* 2006;166:1716–1722.

66. Bradley TD, Logan AG, Kimoff RJ, et al. Continuous positive airway pressure for central sleep apnea and heart failure. *N Engl J Med.* 2005;353:2025–2033.

Chapter 12

Hospital Management of Acute Decompensated Heart Failure

Key Points

- In-hospital and post-discharge mortality of patients hospitalized with decompensated heart failure is high.
- In patients with decompensation of chronic heart failure, typical signs of congestion may not be present on physical examination or chest radiograph.
- Most decompensations are subacute. If a history compatible with symptoms over 24 hours is not present, the patient should be evaluated for other acute exacerbating factors.
- For patients with worsening congestion, diuretic therapy must be rapidly optimized to overcome diuretic resistance.
- Vasodilators can be used in combination with diuretic therapy for rapid relief of dyspnea in patients with systolic blood pressure higher than 100 mmHg.
- Positive inotropic agents should only be used in patients who have clinical manifestations of poor tissue perfusion.
- Discharge planning should include a multidisciplinary assessment to reduce the risk for early readmission.

Clinical Assessment

The term "acute decompensated heart failure" is most often used to describe the change in symptoms leading to hospitalization for heart failure. This term is a misnomer, as multiple lines of evidence indicate that it is a subacute deterioration over one to two weeks that typically leads to hospitalization, although the patient may not perceive any early symptoms of worsening.[1] Regardless of the timing, hospitalization for worsening symptoms of heart failure is a sentinel event that identifies patients at increased risk for post-discharge adverse clinical outcomes.[2]

The decision to hospitalize a patient for worsening symptoms is based primarily on the severity of the symptoms (dyspnea at rest or with minimal exertion, or other persistent symptoms associated with volume overload), identification of precipitating factors or associated conditions that require hospitalization for management, or other factors such as abnormal laboratory values that require hospitalization for safe management.[3] While hospital emergency departments remain the most common destination for patients with decompensated heart failure, other venues, including outpatient furosemide-infusion centers and non-inpatient heart failure observation units, may be suitable alternatives for some patients.[4]

Precipitating factors can be identified in a large proportion of patients with worsening symptoms.[5] Hospitalized patients should be carefully questioned about the events of the two weeks prior to admission, since a precipitating event may be identified in that wider time window. The patient should be questioned about specific potential precipitants, including manifestations of infection, arrhythmias, myocardial ischemia, diuretic resistance, as well as non-compliance with medications and/or sodium restricted diet. It is important to recognize that identification of medicine or dietary non-compliance in the history may not represent a change from usual patient behavior, so this may not necessarily be playing a causal role in the worsening symptoms.

Acute cardiogenic pulmonary edema is a distinct form of decompensated heart failure that is characterized by the sudden onset of severe dyspnea with no prodrome and, in most cases, severe pulmonary venous congestion and alveolar edema with little or no evidence of right-sided congestion. The pathophysiology of acute pulmonary edema is related to acute changes in left-ventricular function, usually due to a combination of myocardial ischemia and sympathetic activation with intense vasoconstriction and consequent high systemic vascular resistance (increased afterload) and increased venous return from displacement of blood from the sphlanchnic circulation (increased preload).[6] Left-ventricular ejection fraction is often normal after initial treatment and return of blood pressure to the normal range.[7] Supraventricular arrhythmia may precipitate acute pulmonary edema in patients with heart failure and preserved ejection fraction. Acute valvular regurgitation lesions and acute myocarditis are also in the differential diagnosis.[8] Although the initiating stimulus cannot be determined in all cases, the final common pathway appears to be an acute rise in pulmonary venous pressures that increases hydrostatic forces in the pulmonary capillaries and causes transudation into the alveolar spaces.[6,9] The evaluation of patients should include search for potential precipitating causes, including ischemia and arrhythmias. Since total body sodium and water content may be normal or only modestly increased, vasodilator therapy (most often intravenous nitroglycerin and opiates) should be the first-line therapy, with additional diuretics as suggested by the physical assessment and response to vasodilators. Ventilator support with continuous positive-pressure breathing or non-invasive positive-pressure ventilation is recommended to reduce the risk of need for tracheal intubation.[10]

In patients presenting with subacute onset of worsening symptoms, physical examination should be directed to determine the volume status of the patient ("wet vs. dry") and evidence of hypoperfusion due to low cardiac output ("warm vs. cold") as described in previous chapters.[3] Pulse and blood pressure should be measured directly by the physician rather than transcribed from nursing notes. Low pulse pressure, thready pulse, and pulsus alternans are consistent with low cardiac output and are often present in patients with reduced ejection fraction. Conversely, hypertension is common is patients with preserved ejection fraction. Respiration should be observed for several minutes to detect cyclic changes in respiratory rate (Cheynes-Stokes respiration). In subacute decompensated heart failure, the absence of rales on lung auscultation does not reliably exclude a cardiac cause of dyspnea (negative predictive value of about 50%).[11] In the absence of inspiratory rales, diffusely decreased bronchial breath sounds are a common physical finding on lung auscultation in patients with acute decompensated heart failure that is consistent with a cardiac cause of dyspnea. Elevation of jugular venous pressures with hepatojugular reflux is the most reliable sign on physical examination. Gallop rhythms are common: S3 gallop in patients with reduced ejection fraction, and S4 gallop in patients with preserved ejection fraction. Other findings of right-sided congestion (hepatomegaly and pre-sacral and/or lower-extremity edema) are common in patients with preserved or reduced ejection fraction.[12,13] Physical examination should also be directed towards identifying potential exacerbation factors such as new or changed cardiac murmur, signs of infection, or thyroid disease.

Chest radiograph is useful to evaluate pulmonary vascular congestion and for evidence of lung infection. In patients with severe hypoxemia and no evidence of infiltrate on chest radiograph, the diagnosis of pulmonary embolism should be considered. Most patients with a subacute presentation will not manifest pulmonary edema on the chest radiography, but may have evidence of pulmonary vascular congestion, small pleural effusions, and Kerley B lines. The absence of such findings does not reliably exclude decompensated heart failure (negative predictive value of chest radiograph for excluding high pulmonary capillary wedge pressure is about 50%).[14] Electrocardiography is useful to evaluate for arrhythmia and ischemia, and for identification of patients with QRS duration >150 msec who may benefit from cardiac resynchronization therapy.

Routine laboratory data can identify exacerbating factors, including elevated white blood cell count, anemia, and worsening renal function. Increase in BUN and serum creatinine levels from previous baseline is consistent with reduced renal perfusion and identifies patients at increased risk for adverse outcomes, but does not provide reliable assessment of intravascular volume.[2] Thyroid function tests are reasonable to exclude hypo- or hyperthyroidism as an exacerbating factor. Abnormal liver function tests (any combination of elevated transaminases and/or hyperbilirubinemia) may be present in patients with evidence of right-heart failure, especially if there is significant tricuspid regurgitation (as detected by presence of an enlarged pulsatile liver on palpation of the abdominal right upper quadrant). In the absence of signs of acute biliary obstruction or other evidence of active liver disease, it is reasonable to defer additional workup unless blood test abnormalities fail to improve after decongestion therapy. Urinalysis should be obtained to evaluate the presence and severity of proteinuria and look for evidence of infection. Fractional excretion of sodium should be low in most cases, but it can be influenced by previous diuretic dosing. A low value is consistent with reduced renal perfusion and does not indicate intravascular volume depletion. As discussed in previous chapters, brain natriuretic peptide measurement can be useful if the volume status of the patient remains uncertain after physical examination and chest radiography.[15]

Confirmatory Testing

Echocardiogram is reasonable to identify changes in ventricular size and function or changes in valve function that may be causally associated with worsening symptoms. Right-heart catheterization is not recommended for routine management of patients with decompensated heart failure.[16] If the patient does not respond to empirical therapy based on clinical assessment as described below, right-heart catheterization may yield information that could be useful for further optimization of therapy.

Risk Assessment

Hospitalized patients presenting with evidence of organ hypoperfusion are at greatest risk for in-hospital death. In a large registry of patients hospitalized with acute decompensated heart failure, the combination of blood pressure <115 mmHg, BUN >40 mg/dl, and serum creatinine >2.5 mg/dl on admission was associated with an in-hospital mortality rate greater than 20%.[2] The occurrence of acute worsening of renal function during the hospitalization (increase in serum creatinine ≥0.3 mg/dl) is also associated with increased risk of in-hospital and post-discharge mortality.[17] Hyponatremia is independently associated with risk of increased in-hospital and post-discharge adverse outcomes in hospitalized patients with heart failure.[18] Increased brain natriuretic peptide levels is also an independent predictor of increased risk of adverse outcomes. The combination of hyponatremia and high brain natriuretic peptide level is associated with the greatest mortality risk.[19]

Treatment Strategies

All patients with acute decompensated heart failure should initially receive treatment with supplemental oxygen, by nasal cannula, or by positive-pressure breathing in patients with pulmonary edema and severe respiratory distress.[20] Severe arterial hypoxemia is not typical of most subacute exacerbations of chronic heart failure, and, if present, it should raise suspicion for coexisting acute lung disease (pneumonia or pulmonary embolism), chronic lung disease, or, more rarely, intracardiac or extracardiac shunts. All patients admitted with decompensated heart failure should receive venous thromboembolism prophylaxis according to institutional protocol.[21]

Most hospitalized patients have a history of chronic heart failure and are receiving chronic medical therapy.[5] Outpatient doses of neurohormonal antagonist therapy (beta-adrenergic-receptor blockers, angiotensin-converting-enzyme inhibitors, angiotensin-receptor blockers, mineralocorticoid-receptor antagonists) should be continued without change in most patients admitted with decompensated heart failure.[17,22] If hypotension (systolic blood pressure <100 mmHg or >20 mmHg below previous baseline), evidence of organ hypoperfusion, and/or worsening renal function are present, neurohormonal antagonists may be discontinued or administered at reduced doses. If neurohormonal antagonist therapy is interrupted or reduced during the hospitalization, therapy should be resumed prior to discharge if possible.

The large majority of patients admitted with decompensated heart failure are classified as "warm" (adequate organ perfusion) and "wet" (signs and symptoms of congestion).[23] The primary therapeutic goal in this subset is effective decongestion therapy. The effectiveness of decongestion therapy should be monitored by patient symptoms, daily weights, daily physical examinations, and daily laboratory evaluations. A summary of the therapeutic approach for decongestion therapy is provided in Figure 12.1. Most patients with chronic heart failure are treated with daily doses of loop diuretics, so a therapeutic strategy must be designed to overcome resistance to the home diuretic regimen.[24] Diuretic resistance is partly attributable to altered gastrointestinal absorption of oral furosemide in response to sphlanchnic congestion.[25,26] Furosemide is absorbed slowly in this setting, with consequent longer time to peak level, lower peak blood level, reduced secretion into the nephron, and diminished pharmacological effect. Patients compliant with their usual daily dose of oral furosemide will frequently report that the diuretic effect was progressively diminished in the weeks before admission. Diuretic resistance is also partly attributable to diminished action of loop diuretics in the renal tubule, in part due to diminished secretion of active drug into the nephron caused by increased competition with endogenous organic acids (such as uric acid), increased reabsorption of sodium in proximal and distal segments of the nephron, and diminished renal blood flow due to low cardiac output and tubuloglomerular feedback. The most commonly applied approach to overcome diuretic resistance is to use intravenous diuretics at higher doses than previous outpatient exposure. A simple rule of thumb for a starting diuretic dose during a hospitalization for decompensation is to administer intravenous furosemide (or equivalent doses of torsemide or bumetanide) at a dose double that of the outpatient daily dose, at 12-hour intervals. The DOSE study demonstrated the safety of this approach in patients hospitalized with heart failure.[27] The response to the initial dose of diuretic should be assessed either by asking the patient if they have noted a large increase in urinary volume, by tracking urine output (although these data are often inaccurate outside of critical care settings), or by sending a spot urine sample for urinary sodium 1–2 hours after intravenous administration of the diuretic. An effective dose of diuretic should increase urine output to >200 ml/hr for several hours with urinary sodium content >100 meq/l. If the initial selected diuretic dose does not achieve these goals, the next dose should be doubled (to a maximum of 240 mg intravenous administration every 12 hours). For most patients, a net negative fluid balance of 1–2 liters per day (corresponding to decreased weight of 1–2 kg/day) is a reasonable goal for diuretic therapy. For patients with more severe volume overload (known to be >10kg over their previous baseline weight, or the presence of edema above the knees, or ascites), a goal weight loss of 2–3 kg/day is appropriate. To minimize the risk of ototoxicity, the rate of administration of intravenous furosemide should be reduced for doses >80 mg (maximum 10 mg/min). A continuous furosemide infusion can be considered in patients with evidence of severe volume overload (edema above the knees and/or ascites), although the DOSE study demonstrated no difference in efficacy or safety between intravenous bolus vs. continuous infusion of furosemide.[27] The infusion rate can be adjusted to achieve a net fluid loss of 2–3 liters per day as tolerated. A downside of the continuous-infusion approach is limitation of patient mobility (and increased fall risk) due to the need for an infusion pump and intravenous pump stand. Patients receiving intravenous loop diuretics are at risk for hypokalemia, so they should preemptively receive oral potassium chloride supplementation at the time of initiation of therapy. In patients with estimated glomerular filtration rate >30 ml/min and serum potassium <5.0 meq/l, a starting dose of potassium chloride 40 meq twice daily is reasonable, with adjustment based on serial laboratory testing. Spot urinary potassium levels can be used to calculate urinary potassium losses in the setting of severely impaired renal function or history of hyperkalemia. An added benefit of aggressive potassium chloride supplementation is amelioration of the hypochloremic metabolic alkalosis associated with diuretic therapy. Potassium chloride supplementation is the treatment of first choice in the setting of hypochloremic metabolic alkalosis, unless the serum potassium level is >5.0 meq/l. In patients on higher doses of mineralocorticoid receptor antagonists and/or serum potassium >5.0 meq/l, acetazolamide 250 mg four times daily can be administered for several days to increase diuresis and raise serum chloride levels.[28]

Patients who do not respond to high-dose intravenous loop diuretics are at higher risk for prolonged hospitalization, worsening renal function during the hospitalization, and in-hospital and post-discharge adverse clinical outcomes. Addition of a thiazide diuretic (oral hydrochlorothiazide 12.5 mg–50 mg or intravenous chlorothiazide 500 mg daily) or thiazide-like diuretic (oral metolazone 2.5 mg–10 mg daily) is an effective strategy to overcome diuretic resistance and increase urine output.[29] A single-dose order for initiation of therapy is recommended, as the response to combination therapy is unpredictable, and in some patients can it induce a sustained, large increase in urinary volume (>300 ml/hr) with associated hypokalemia, hypomagnesiumia, hypovolemia, and hypotension. Administration 30 minutes before intravenous loop diuretic dosing is not required. Once the 24-hour response to the first dose has been assessed, the dose and dosing interval of the agent can be adjusted, remembering that the half-life of thiazide diuretics is substantially longer than that of loop diuretics. Oral potassium chloride supplementation should be increased in patients

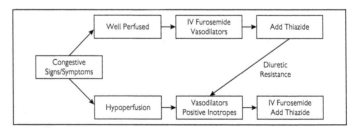

Figure 12.1 Therapeutic strategies based on clinical presentation in patients with hospitalized with worsening heart failure. (See chapter text for details.)

receiving combination diuretic therapy with careful monitoring of electrolytes and addition of magnesium supplementation as needed.

For patients resistant to combination diuretic therapy, ultrafiltration therapy can be considered. This technique requires central intravenous access and systemic heparinization, but has been shown to be a safe and effective means of reducing congestion in patients hospitalized with decompensated heart failure. Potential advantages of the ultrafiltration approach vs. loop diuretics include a greater concentration of sodium removal in the ultrafiltrate compared with urine, and reduced potassium losses. However, the risk of worsening of renal function associated with decongestion therapy via ultrafiltration is not lower than the risk associated with decongestion therapy with loop diuretics.[30,31]

For patients with evidence of low cardiac output and renal hypoperfusion, positive inotropic therapy with dobutamine or milrinone may be considered in order to improve renal perfusion and enhance response to diuretics.[32] Dopamine administered at low doses (1–3 mcg/kg/min) selectively increases renal blood flow and in some patients can enhance the response to loop diuretics.[33] Dopamine should be not be administered via a peripheral intravenous line, since extravasation could lead to a serious local skin tissue injury (due to severe vasoconstriction).

Most patients treated with decongestion therapy (diuretics and/or ultrafiltration) will demonstrate an increase in serum creatinine in response to therapy. This increase in serum creatinine in the setting of treatment of decompensated heart failure is one manifestation of a larger group of disorders collectively called *cardiorenal syndrome*.[34] The pathophysiology of the worsening of renal function in response to decongestion therapy is complex and heterogeneous, but can be attributed to systemic hemodynamic changes, renal hemodynamic changes, and other intrarenal changes in response to decongestion. One of the principal goals of decongestion therapy is to reduce ventricular preload. In most patients with heart failure with reduced ejection fraction, preload reduction is not associated with reduction of cardiac output, unless the pulmonary capillary wedge pressure decreases to below 12 mmHg. The likelihood of excessive reduction in preload is low for most patients with reduced ejection fraction, but it may be more likely in patients with very rapid diuresis rate (one that exceeds capillary refill rate from the extravascular tissues) and low plasma oncotic pressure due to nephrotic syndrome, cardiac cachexia with malnutrition, or chronic liver disease. Conversely, patients with heart failure and preserved ejection fraction may more often manifest a decrease in forward cardiac output (and decreased renal perfusion) in response to preload reduction with diuretic therapy. Despite the effects of reduced preload on cardiac output in some patients, any reduction in net perfusion gradient across the renal circulation associated with reduced arterial pressure is partially offset by concomitant reduction in systemic venous pressures in response to diuretic therapy. In addition to the effects of decongestion therapy on the pressure gradient across the kidney circulation, neurohormonal activation in response to reduced cardiac output can alter glomerular hemodynamics and decrease renal arterial blood flow. Increased delivery of sodium to the macula densa in response to loop diuretics can further decrease renal blood flow and glomerular filtration. All of these mechanisms can contribute to rising creatinine, but they are not typically associated with renal tubular injury or oliguria. Loop diuretics are known to decrease renal oxygen consumption and reduce the extent of tubular injury in experimental models of renal ischemia.[35,36] Accordingly, acute oliguric renal failure with evidence of acute tubular necrosis is unlikely to be directly attributable to loop diuretic therapy. Lastly, in patients with a large volume of diuresis during therapy (>10 kg weight loss), total body sodium and water may be reduced by 10%–20% with consequent increased concentration of serum creatinine that is unrelated to change in glomerular filtration rate.

Worsening renal function during hospitalization for decompensated heart failure (increase in creatinine >0.3 mg/dl) has been shown to be associated with increased risk of in-hospital and post-discharge mortality. Higher diuretic doses have also been associated with greater risk of adverse outcomes.[17] However, successful decongestion therapy (as evidenced by weight reduction and hemoconcentration, an increase in hematocrit, serum albumin, and/or total protein during the hospitalization) is associated with reduced risk of post-discharge mortality despite worsening renal function during treatment.[37,38] The DOSE study confirmed that patients randomly assigned to higher doses of diuretics during hospitalization for decompensated heart failure demonstrated greater weight loss, increased risk of worsening function, but no evidence of increased risk of post-discharge adverse clinical outcomes when compared with patients randomized to lower doses of diuretics.[27]

Taking into account the complex pathophysiology and data on clinical outcomes described above, it is recommended to adjust diuretic therapy primarily based on the clinical assessment of cardiac filling pressures (most reliably, jugular venous pressure waves) rather than on blood pressure, blood urea nitrogen levels, or serum creatinine levels. If the patient has clear evidence of persistent elevation of jugular venous pressures (>8 cm above the angle of Louis), diuretic or ultrafiltration therapy should continue with a goal of achieving resolution of congestive signs and symptoms. If the signs of congestion persist in conjunction with signs of reduced perfusion ("cold and wet"), then additional therapy should be considered to improve renal perfusion as described below. These therapies should be administered in hospital setting able to provide frequent monitoring of patients (intensive care or step-down units, per institutional protocol).

Vasodilator therapy can be used in conjunction with diuretic therapy for symptom relief in patients with evidence of congestion and systolic blood pressure >100 mmHg ("warm and wet"). Intravenous nitroglycerin has a short serum half-life and can be rapidly titrated to a typical target range of 100–400 mcg/min as dictated by systemic blood pressure and signs and symptoms of congestion.[39] Intravenous nitroglycerin can be especially helpful in patients with functional mitral regurgitation due to mitral annular dilatation. Nitroglycerin rapidly reduces preload, with concomitant decrease in regurgitant volume and increased forward cardiac output in this subset of patients.[40] Nitroglycerin's hemodynamic effects can rapidly diminish over 24 hours.[41] Short-term use is usually sufficient to achieve early treatment goals, but if longer duration of therapy is planned, the therapeutic effect must be reassessed daily with further up-titration as necessary. Some patients with initial good response to nitroglycerin may eventually become resistant to its vasodilating effects. Nesiritide is an alternative vasodilator agent that is suitable for longer term use, as rapid toler-ance has not been described with this agent.[42]

Patients with reduced ejection fraction and evidence of congestion and peripheral hypoperfusion ("wet and cold") may be managed with vasodilators as described above if the systolic blood pressure is >100 mmHg, or positive inotropic agents if the systolic blood pressure is < 100 mmHg. Dobutamine and milrinone can be used to increase cardiac output as described in Chapter 10. Positive inotropic agents have been associated with increased risk of adverse clinical outcomes in clinical trials of hospitalized heart failure patients (with or without evidence of low cardiac output), but the safety of these agents in the specific situation of treatment of low-cardiac-output syndrome has never been tested prospectively. An observational registry of a large number of patients hospitalized with decompensated heart failure suggested that the use of posi-tive inotropic agents is associated with increased risk of adverse outcomes, even when adjusting for severity of illness.[43] Given these safety concerns, the goal for use of positive inotropic agents is to use the lowest possible dose for the shortest period of time to return the patient to a compensated state with optimal volume status.

Length of hospital stay can be minimized by hospital-wide programs to increase early and accurate recognition of heart failure patients, and by develop-ment of treatment protocols and order sets to assist in the rapid titration of diuretic dose.[44] The DOSE study has confirmed the safety of higher initial doses of intravenous diuretics (twice the outpatient oral diuretic dose) in hospitalized patients with signs and symptoms of congestion.[27] The pathophysiology of heart failure is too complex to create a formulaic approach for all patients. The treat-ment plan must be individualized with an emphasis on the frequent assessments of clinical response to therapy with appropriate adjustments of the medical regimen as needed.

The goal of the initial treatment strategies described above is to relieve symptoms associated with decompensation, address any identified exacerbating factors, and restore the patient to a stable clinical state for transition back to oral therapies and discharge from the hospital. For discharge to home, patients should demonstrate ability to ambulate at their preadmission level and perform simple activities of daily living (bathing, dressing) without symptoms. Patients unable to perform these tasks may not be suitable for home discharge, and may benefit from transfer to acute or subacute rehabilitation facilities. Early consultation with physiatry and physical therapy services will aid in determina-tion of the optimal discharge venue. The final day(s) of the hospital course should be used to optimize outpatient therapy.[45] If the initial presentation was predominantly due to volume overload ("warm and wet"), outpatient diuretic dosing should be reevaluated at the time of discharge. For patients with recur-rent admissions, it is reasonable to consider an increase of the furosemide dose, or a change to torsemide, as the oral bioavailability of this agent may be supe-rior to that of furosemide in some patients.[46] If doses of neurohormonal agents were held or reduced during the course of the hospitalization, the medications should be reviewed, and if possible restarted and/or increased back to admis-sion doses.[45] The therapeutic regimen should be reviewed to determine that the patient is receiving all indicated medical and device therapy. A multidisciplinary plan should be developed to address cardiovascular issues, non-cardiovascular issues, and psychosocial issues pertinent for each patient. The discharge planning process and transition to care outside the hospital is described in detail in Chapter 13.

References

1. Desai AS, Stevenson LW. Rehospitalization for heart failure: predict or prevent? *Circulation*. 2012;126:501–506.

2. Fonarow GC, Adams KF, Jr., Abraham WT, Yancy CW, Boscardin WJ. Risk stratification for in-hospital mortality in acutely decompensated heart failure: classification and regression tree analysis. *JAMA*. 2005;293:572–580.

3. Thomas SS, Nohria A. Hemodynamic classifications of acute heart failure and their clinical application—an update. *Circ J*. 2012;76:278–286.

4. Peacock WF 4th, Young J, Collins S, Diercks D, Emerman C. Heart failure observation units: optimizing care. *Ann Emerg Med*. 2006;47:22–33.

5. Klapholz M, Maurer M, Lowe AM, et al. Hospitalization for heart failure in the presence of a normal left-ventricular ejection fraction: results of the New York Heart Failure Registry. *J Am Coll Cardiol*. 2004;43:1432–1438.

6. Luisada AA, Cardi L. Acute pulmonary edema; pathology, physiology and clinical management. *Circulation*. 1956;13:113–135.

7. Gandhi SK, Powers JC, Nomeir AM, et al. The pathogenesis of acute pulmonary edema associated with hypertension. *N Engl J Med*. 2001;344:17–22.

8. Pierard LA, Lancellotti P. The role of ischemic mitral regurgitation in the pathogenesis of acute pulmonary edema. *N Engl J Med*. 2004;351:1627–1634.

9. Ware LB, Matthay MA. Clinical practice. Acute pulmonary edema. *N Engl J Med*. 2005;353:2788–2796.

10. Mehta S. Continuous versus bilevel positive airway pressure in acute cardiogenic pulmonary edema? A good question! *Crit Care Med*. 2004;32:2546–2548.

11. Butman SM, Ewy GA, Standen JR, Kern KB, Hahn E. Bedside cardiovascular examination in patients with severe chronic heart failure: importance of rest or inducible jugular venous distension. *J Am Coll Cardiol*. 1993;22:968–974.

12. Fonarow GC, Heywood JT, Heidenreich PA, Lopatin M, Yancy CW; Committee ASA investigators. Temporal trends in clinical characteristics, treatments, and outcomes for heart failure hospitalizations, 2002 to 2004: findings from Acute Decompensated Heart Failure National Registry (ADHERE). *Am Heart J*. 2007;153:1021–1028.

13. Yancy CW, Lopatin M, Stevenson LW, De Marco T, Fonarow GC. Clinical presentation, management, and in-hospital outcomes of patients admitted with acute decompensated heart failure with preserved systolic function: a report from the Acute Decompensated Heart Failure National Registry (ADHERE) database. *J Am Coll Cardiol*. 2006;47:76–84.

14. Chakko S, Woska D, Martinez H, et al. Clinical, radiographic, and hemodynamic correlations in chronic congestive heart failure: conflicting results may lead to inappropriate care. *Am J Med*. 1991;90:353–359.

15. de Lemos JA, McGuire DK, Drazner MH. B-type natriuretic peptide in cardiovascular disease. *Lancet*. 2003;362:316–322.

16. Binanay C, Califf RM, Hasselblad V, et al. Evaluation study of congestive heart failure and pulmonary artery catheterization effectiveness: the ESCAPE trial. *JAMA*. 2005;294:1625–1633.

17. Damman K, Navis G, Voors AA, et al. Worsening renal function and prognosis in heart failure: Systematic review and meta-analysis. *J Card Fail.* 2007;13:599–608.

18. Gheorghiade M, Rossi JS, Cotts W, et al. Characterization and prognostic value of persistent hyponatremia in patients with severe heart failure in the ESCAPE trial. *Arch Intern Med.* 2007;167:1998–2005.

19. Mohammed AA, van Kimmenade RR, Richards M, et al. Hyponatremia, natriuretic peptides, and outcomes in acutely decompensated heart failure: results from the International Collaborative of NT-PROBNP study. *Circ. Heart Fail.* 2010;3:354–361.

20. Tallman TA, Peacock WF, Emerman CL, et al. Noninvasive ventilation outcomes in 2,430 acute decompensated heart failure patients: an ADHERE Registry analysis. *Acad Emerg Med.* 2008;15:355–362.

21. Jois-Bilowich P, Michota F, Bartholomew JR, et al.; ADHERE Scientific Advisory C investigators. Venous thromboembolism prophylaxis in hospitalized heart failure patients. *J Card Fail.* 2008;14:127–132.

22. Jondeau G, Neuder Y, Eicher JC, et al. B-convinced: beta-blocker continuation vs. interruption in patients with congestive heart failure hospitalized for a decompensation episode. *Eur Heart J.* 2009;30:2186–2192.

23. Nohria A, Tsang SW, Fang JC, et al. Clinical assessment identifies hemodynamic profiles that predict outcomes in patients admitted with heart failure. *J Am Coll Cardiol.* 2003;41:1797–1804.

24. Brater DC. Diuretic therapy. *N Engl J Med.* 1998;339:387–395.

25. Gottlieb SS, Khatta M, Wentworth D, Roffman D, Fisher ML, Kramer WG. The effects of diuresis on the pharmacokinetics of the loop diuretics furosemide and torsemide in patients with heart failure. *Am J Med.* 1998;104:533–538.

26. Vasko MR, Cartwright DB, Knochel JP, Nixon JV, Brater DC. Furosemide absorption altered in decompensated congestive heart failure. *Ann Intern Med.* 1985;102:314–318.

27. Felker GM, Lee KL, Bull DA, et al. Diuretic strategies in patients with acute decompensated heart failure. *N Engl J Med.* 2011;364:797–805.

28. Khan MI. Treatment of refractory congestive heart failure and normokalemic hypochloremic alkalosis with acetazolamide and spironolactone. *CMAJ.* 1980;123:883–887.

29. Rosenberg J, Gustafsson F, Galatius S, Hildebrandt PR. Combination therapy with metolazone and loop diuretics in outpatients with refractory heart failure: an observational study and review of the literature. *Cardiovasc Drugs Ther.* 2005;19:301–306.

30. Bart BA, Goldsmith SR, Lee KL, et al. Ultrafiltration in decompensated heart failure with cardiorenal syndrome. *N Engl J Med.* 2012;367:2296–2304.

31. Costanzo MR, Guglin ME, Saltzberg MT, et al. Ultrafiltration versus intravenous diuretics for patients hospitalized for acute decompensated heart failure. *J Am Coll Cardiol.* 2007;49:675–683.

32. Anderson JL, Baim DS, Fein SA, Goldstein RA, LeJemtel TH, Likoff MJ. Efficacy and safety of sustained (48-hour) intravenous infusions of milrinone in patients with severe congestive heart failure: a multicenter study. *J Am Coll Cardiol.* 1987;9:711–722.

33. Maskin CS, Ocken S, Chadwick B, LeJemtel TH. Comparative systemic and renal effects of dopamine and angiotensin-converting enzyme inhibition with enalaprilat in patients with heart failure. *Circulation.* 1985;72:846–852.

34. Damman K, Voors AA, Navis G, van Veldhuisen DJ, Hillege HL. The cardiorenal syndrome in heart failure. *Prog Cardiovasc Dis.* 2011;54:144–153.

35. Brezis M, Rosen S. Hypoxia of the renal medulla—its implications for disease. *N Engl J Med.* 1995;332:647–655.

36. Heyman SN, Rosen S, Epstein FH, Spokes K, Brezis ML. Loop diuretics reduce hypoxic damage to proximal tubules of the isolated perfused rat kidney. *Kidney Int.* 1994;45:981–985.

37. Davila C, Reyentovich A, Katz SD. Clinical correlates of hemoconcentration during hospitalization for acute decompensated heart failure. *J Card Fail.* 2011;17:1018–1022.

38. Testani JM, Chen J, McCauley BD, Kimmel SE, Shannon RP. Potential effects of aggressive decongestion during the treatment of decompensated heart failure on renal function and survival. *Circulation.* 2010;122:265–272.

39. Intravenous nesiritide vs. nitroglycerin for treatment of decompensated congestive heart failure: a randomized controlled trial. *JAMA.* 2002;287:1531–1540.

40. Keren G, Katz S, Strom J, Sonnenblick EH, LeJemtel TH. Dynamic mitral regurgitation. An important determinant of the hemodynamic response to load alterations and inotropic therapy in severe heart failure. *Circulation.* 1989;80:306–313.

41. Packer M, Lee WH, Kessler PD, Gottlieb SS, Medina N, Yushak M. Prevention and reversal of nitrate tolerance in patients with congestive heart failure. *N Engl J Med.* 1987;317:799–804.

42. O'Connor CM, Starling RC, Hernandez AF, et al. Effect of nesiritide in patients with acute decompensated heart failure. *N Engl J Med.* 2011;365:32–43.

43. Abraham WT, Adams KF, Fonarow GC, et al. In-hospital mortality in patients with acute decompensated heart failure requiring intravenous vasoactive medications: an analysis from the Acute Decompensated Heart Failure National Registry (ADHERE). *J Am Coll Cardiol.* 2005;46:57–64.

44. Felker GM, O'Connor CM, Braunwald E, Heart Failure Clinical Research Network I. Loop diuretics in acute decompensated heart failure: Necessary? Evil? A necessary evil? *Circ. Heart Fail.* 2009;2:56–62.

45. Gattis WA, O'Connor CM, Gallup DS, Hasselblad V, Gheorghiade M, Investigators I-H, coordinators. Predischarge initiation of carvedilol in patients hospitalized for decompensated heart failure: results of the Initiation Management Predischarge: Process for Assessment of Carvedilol Therapy in Heart Failure (IMPACT-HF) trial. *J Am Coll Cardiol.* 2004;43:1534–1541.

46. Vargo DL, Kramer WG, Black PK, Smith WB, Serpas T, Brater DC. Bioavailability, pharmacokinetics, and pharmacodynamics of torsemide and furosemide in patients with congestive heart failure. *Clin Pharmacol Ther.* 1995;57:601–609.

Chapter 13

Transitions of Care

Key Points

- *Transitional care* refers to the aspects of health care designed to optimize coordination of the care plan at the time of a change in location or care providers.
- Patients hospitalized for heart failure have a high rate of post-discharge re-hospitalization (approximately 25% at 30 days) and mortality (33% at one year).
- Community-based multidisciplinary programs (disease management combined with case management) with face-to-face communication appear to be most consistently associated with reduction of adverse outcomes in patients with recent hospitalization for heart failure.
- Referral to specialized heart failure centers with team care capability should be considered in patients with recurrent hospitalizations or high-risk comorbidities.
- Optimization of care according to evidenced-based guidelines has been shown to be associated with improved clinical outcomes.
- Shared decision-making based on a dialogue between provider and patient is necessary to determine the appropriate goals of care in patients with heart failure.

"Transitional care" refers to the aspects of health care designed to optimize coordination of the care plan at the time of a change in location or care providers.[1] Effective transitional care depends on adequate communication between in-hospital providers (physician and non-physician), post-discharge care providers (physician and non-physician), the patient, and the patient's caregivers (family members, companions, and/or professional home-care providers). There are many systemic barriers to implementation of effective transitional care, including increasing fragmentation of care with multiple providers (both inpatient and post-discharge), lack of connectivity between inpatient and outpatient medical records, and reduced length of hospital stay. Heart failure patients offer special challenges for effective transitional care due to the high prevalence of multiple comorbidities and complex polypharmacy regimen in many patients.

Patients hospitalized for heart failure have a high rate of post-discharge re-hospitalization (approximately 25% at 30 days) and mortality (33% at one year).[2–4] Fewer than 2% of patients survive more than 10 years after an index heart failure hospitalization. Recurrent hospitalizations are clustered in the first few months after an index hospitalization and in the last few months of life.[4,5] Since hospitalization is a major determinant of the high healthcare costs associated with heart failure, reduction of recurrent hospitalizations has been selected as a quality performance measure with substantial impact on future hospital reimbursements. The potential loss of revenues associated with hospital readmissions in the heart failure population has spurred interest among hospital administrators for development of hospital-based outreach programs to reduce readmission risk. Programs designed to reduce readmission are based on the premise that a certain proportion of readmissions are preventable. Available data suggest that many of the hospital admissions may not be truly preventable (and in fact are beneficial for patients), and thus should not be eliminated by specific disease-management or care-management programs.[5] Non-cardiac admission diagnoses make up a large proportion of the re-hospitalizations and thus may not be impacted by disease management programs directed at optimization of heart failure therapy. Re-hospitalization rates are known to vary across the United States by geographic region, and in part, appear to be determined by regional variations in the clinical characteristics of the heart failure population and the availability of hospital and non-hospital health care resources in the community.[6]

Risk factors for re-hospitalization and mortality after heart failure hospitalization have been assessed in numerous studies. However, the reported results are largely inconsistent and have not yielded a consensus on a validated risk-assessment model for application in clinical practice.[5,7] Accordingly, each hospitalized heart failure patient must be considered to be at high risk for adverse outcomes, and therefore may benefit from a coordinated effort to optimize the transition of care at the time of hospital discharge.

The transition process may be categorized according to the location of care (in hospital vs. community care), type of care providers (physicians, nurses, and other ancillary personnel), and method of communication (face-to-face vs. phone or Internet).[3,8] Programs can be further organized, with components of disease management (optimization of heart failure therapy according to evidence-based practice guidelines with ongoing assessment of program impact on patient outcomes) and case management (facilitation of community-based health-related and social services and facilitation of communication among health care providers). The optimal strategy for reduction of adverse outcomes has not been determined.[9] Community-based multidisciplinary programs (disease management combined with case management) with face-to-face communication appear to be most consistently associated with reduction of adverse outcomes. The cost-effectiveness of this labor-intensive approach has not been determined. Use of centralized telemonitoring with customized algorithms that trigger face-to-face meetings from a multidisciplinary team member when needed may be a more cost-effective strategy.[10] The strategy must be customized according to the available resources of each institution, geographical considerations, and the needs of each patient within the institution. In-hospital and post-discharge care providers must be familiar with the range of services available in the hospital and community, and must be able to effectively communicate with each other and other care providers and ancillary staff to identify the necessary resources for their patient. Since this complex process often takes several days, all heart failure patients should be evaluated by the social work service and/or multidisciplinary case management team at the time of hospital admission. Likely post-discharge disposition (home, acute rehabilitation facility, subacute rehabilitation facility, nursing home facility, home hospice or hospice facility) should be discussed among care providers during the first 24 hours of hospitalization, with appropriate consultations from rehabilitation medicine and, if appropriate, palliative care medicine. For elderly patients with multiple comorbidities, a geriatrics consult is often helpful to address polypharmacy, cognitive dysfunction, depression, and non-cardiac limitations of functional capacity issues (frailty, orthopedic problems, pain, gait disturbance, fall risk) that often contribute to hospital readmission.

During hospitalization, all patients should receive written materials in their native language with information on advance directives, and self-care behaviors for heart failure (daily weights, daily assessment of edema, medication and diet adherence, low level exercise, keeping appointments with health care providers, recognition of worsening symptoms). Healthcare literacy should be assessed in all patients by validated questionnaires or by asking the patient to read a section of the educational material out loud and explain its meaning. Several one-on-one education sessions should be scheduled during the hospitalization to reinforce teaching of these important behaviors. Hospital-based education alone is not sufficient to reduce risk or rehospitalization, so it must be linked to continued education after discharge.[11]

For patients discharged to their home, a follow-up visit with a healthcare provider within three to seven days of discharge is recommended in order to identify problems with filling of discharge medication prescriptions, or any misunderstanding about the home medical regimen, and to identify signs and symptoms of rapid destabilization of the patient. This early post-discharge visit is also an important opportunity to discuss advance directives and review self-management behaviors. In response to the recognition of the high risk of recurrent hospitalization in the heart failure population (and the potential loss of revenues associated with re-hospitalization), hospital-based employees may play a greater role in post-discharge care in the future. Nursing staff and case management staff can optimize the transitional care through integration with outpatient medical office personnel to effectively communicate changes in medical regimens, provide patient and office staff education, and assess needs for home care services.

Patients with multiple hospital readmissions or multiple high-risk comorbidities (chronic lung disease, chronic kidney disease) may benefit from referral to a specialized heart failure clinic. Specialized heart failure centers differ from most non-specialized practice settings by providing a team-based approach to patient management by physicians and nurses with special training and experience in heart failure and a higher provider–patient ratio.[12,13] Specialized heart failure centers should be staffed with expert physician and nursing providers to optimize disease management, recognize and manage cognitive dysfunction and depression, provide ongoing education to promote patient self-management behaviors and adherence to the prescribed medical regimen, and increase accessibility to care, with flexible schedules for urgent visits. Specialized heart failure centers can also provide expert assessment of patients with advanced disease to determine which patients may benefit from advanced therapies such as electrophysiological devices or procedures, mechanical circulatory support devices, and cardiac transplantation. While these services offered by heart failure clinics appear to provide clinical benefits to some patients, there is no evidence that specialized heart failure center referral reduces mortality or re-hospitalization risk.[14] However, optimization of medical and device therapy according to evidence-based guideline recommendations has been reported to be associated with improved clinical outcomes in a real-world setting.[15]

Hospitalization for heart failure identifies patients at high risk for subsequent mortality after discharge. Accordingly, an index hospitalization should prompt initiation of discussions for shared decision-making.[16] Shared decision-making is an integral component of patient-centered care, and is based on frank dialogues between care providers and the patient (and patient-designated family members or companions) with regard to goals of care. The care provider must use clinical skills to assess prognosis for both survival and likely quality of life, determine medically appropriate treatment modalities (including no intervention and/or palliative care options), and inform the patients of the risks and benefits of each of these modalities. It is important that the provider acknowledge the inherent uncertainty of their assessment with regard to prognosis and response to treatment. The provider should solicit the patients' assessment of their expectations of care based on their understanding of their disease and the information received. Discussions of goals of care are often difficult to initiate in busy clinical practices with limited time allotted for each visit. Scheduling a longer annual visit to discuss goals of care is a reasonable approach that may be carried out within the primary care practice, or in conjunction with a specialized heart failure center. Alternatively, an acute hospitalization offers an opportunity to initiate a discussion of advance directives during the hospital stay and schedule post-discharge visits to continue discussion of goals of care in an outpatient setting. Other clinical events that should trigger discussion include the need for higher diuretic doses without obvious change in dietary habits, worsening chronic kidney disease, a shock administered by an implantable cardiovertor-defibrillator, or the need to reduce dose or withdraw neurohormonal antagonists because of new symptomatic hypotension.

In patients with anticipated life expectancy of less than six months, a discussion of end-of-life care options should be initiated by the provider—ideally within the context of ongoing discussions of goals of care initiated earlier in the disease process, as discussed above. Deactivation of implantable cardiovertor-defibrillators, implementation of palliative care therapies, transition from acute hospital to hospice care, and resuscitation preferences should be considered in accordance with patient treatment goals.[17]

References

1. Coleman EA, Berenson RA. Lost in transition: challenges and opportunities for improving the quality of transitional care. *Ann Intern Med.* 2004;141:533–536.

2. Hernandez AF, Greiner MA, Fonarow GC, et al. Relationship between early physician follow-up and 30-day readmission among Medicare beneficiaries hospitalized for heart failure. *JAMA.* 2010;303:1716–1722.

3. Kociol RD, Peterson ED, Hammill BG, et al. National survey of hospital strategies to reduce heart failure readmissions: findings from the Get with the Guidelines–Heart Failure Registry. *Circ. Heart Fail.* 2012;5:680–687.

4. Chun S, Tu JV, Wijeysundera HC, et al. Lifetime analysis of hospitalizations and survival of patients newly admitted with heart failure. *Circ. Heart Fail.* 2012;5:414–421.

5. Desai AS, Stevenson LW. Rehospitalization for heart failure: predict or prevent? *Circulation.* 2012;126:501–506.

6. Joynt KE, Jha AK. Thirty-day readmissions—truth and consequences. *N Engl J Med.* 2012;366:1366–1369.

7. Ross JS, Mulvey GK, Stauffer B, et al. Statistical models and patient predictors of readmission for heart failure: a systematic review. *Arch Intern Med.* 2008;168:1371–1386.

8. Krumholz HM, Currie PM, Riegel B, et al. A taxonomy for disease management: a scientific statement from the American Heart Association Disease Management Taxonomy writing group. *Circulation.* 2006;114:1432–1445.

9. Desai AS. Home monitoring heart failure care does not improve patient outcomes: looking beyond telephone-based disease management. *Circulation.* 2012;125:828–836.

10. Whellan DJ, Hasselblad V, Peterson E, O'Connor CM, Schulman KA. Metaanalysis and review of heart failure disease management randomized controlled clinical trials. *Am Heart J.* 2005;149:722–729.

11. Lainscak M, Blue L, Clark AL, et al. Self-care management of heart failure: practical recommendations from the Patient Care Committee of the Heart Failure Association of the European Society of Cardiology. *Eur J Heart Fail.* 2011;13:115–126.

12. Grady KL, Dracup K, Kennedy G, et al. Team management of patients with heart failure: a statement for healthcare professionals from the Cardiovascular Nursing Council of the American Heart Association. *Circulation.* 2000;102:2443–2456.

13. Hauptman PJ, Rich MW, Heidenreich PA, et al.; Heart Failure Society of America. The heart failure clinic: a consensus statement of the heart Failure Society of America. *J Cardiac Fail.* 2008;14:801–815.

14. Hummel SL, Pauli NP, Krumholz HM, et al. Thirty-day outcomes in Medicare patients with heart failure at heart transplant centers. *Circ. Heart Fail.* 2010;3:244–252.

15. Fonarow GC, Albert NM, Curtis AB, et al. Incremental reduction in risk of death associated with use of guideline-recommended therapies in patients with heart failure: A nested case-control analysis of the Registry to Improve Heart Failure Therapies in the Outpatient Setting (IMPROVE-HF). *JAHA.* 2012;1:16–26.

16. Allen LA, Stevenson LW, Grady KL, et al. Decision-making in advanced heart failure: a scientific statement from the American Heart Association. *Circulation.* 2012;125:1928–1952.

17. Lampert R, Hayes DL, Annas GJ, et al.; endorsed by the American College of Cardiology, the American Geriatrics Society, the American Academy of Hospice and Palliative Medicine, the American Heart Association, the European Heart Rhythm Association, and the Hospice and Palliative Nurses Association. Heart Rhythm Society (HRS) Expert Consensus Statement on the management of cardiovascular implantable electronic devices (CIEDS) in patients nearing end of life or requesting withdrawal of therapy. *Heart Rhythm.* 2010;7:1008–1026.

Appendix: Consensus guidelines for the diagnosis and treatment of heart failure

1. Arnold JM, Liu P, Demers C, Dorian P, Giannetti N, Haddad H, Heckman GA, Howlett JG, Ignaszewski A, Johnstone DE, Jong P, McKelvie RS, Moe GW, Parker JD, Rao V, Ross HJ, Sequeira EJ, Svendsen AM, Teo K, Tsuyuki RT, White M, Canadian Cardiovascular Society. Canadian cardiovascular society consensus conference recommendations on heart failure 2006: Diagnosis and management. *The Canadian journal of cardiology.* 2006;22:23–45.
   Also available at: http://www.ccs.ca/home/index_e.aspx
2. Lindenfeld J, Albert NM, Boehmer JP, Collins SP, Ezekowitz JA, Givertz MM, Katz SD, Klapholz M, Moser DK, Rogers JG, Starling RC, Stevenson WG, Tang WH, Teerlink JR, Walsh MN. Heart Failure Society of America 2010 comprehensive heart failure practice guideline. *Journal of cardiac failure.* 2010;16:e1–194.
   Also available at: http://www.hfsa.org
3. Hunt SA, Abraham WT, Chin MH, Feldman AM, Francis GS, Ganiats TG, Jessup M, Konstam MA, Mancini DM, Michl K, Oates JA, Rahko PS, Silver MA, Stevenson LW, Yancy CW. 2009 focused update incorporated into the American College of Cardiology/American Heart Association 2005 guidelines for the diagnosis and management of heart failure in adults: A report of the American College of Cardiology Foundation/American Heart Association Task Force on practice guidelines: Developed in collaboration with the International Society for Heart and Lung Transplantation. *Circulation.* 2009;119:e391–479.
   Also available at: http://my.americanheart.org/professional/StatementsGuidelines/ByTopic/TopicsD-H/Heart-Failure_UCM_321545_Article.jsp
4. McMurray JJ, Adamopoulos S, Anker SD, Auricchio A, Bohm M, Dickstein K, Falk V, Filippatos G, Fonseca C, Gomez-Sanchez MA, Jaarsma T, Kober L, Lip GY, Maggioni AP, Parkhomenko A, Pieske BM, Popescu BA, Ronnevik PK, Rutten FH, Schwitter J, Seferovic P, Stepinska J, Trindade PT, Voors AA, Zannad F, Zeiher A. European Society of Cardiology guidelines for the diagnosis and treatment of acute and chronic heart failure 2012: The task force for the diagnosis and treatment of acute and chronic heart failure 2012 of the European Society of Cardiology. Developed in

collaboration with the Heart Failure Association of the European Society of Cardiology. *European heart journal*. 2012;33:1787–1847.

Also available at: http://www.escardio.org/guidelines-surveys/esc-guidelines/Pages/acute-chronic-heart-failure.aspx

Index

Page numbers followed by "t" indicate a table and "f" indicate a figure.

Wes
8/20

...one of the
funniest,
most finely achieved comic novels,
even by her own standard ... a masterpiece.'
ALI SMITH

'A timely critique of
political and narrative authority
...
Nicola Barker is
literary royalty
...
The quartet of characters involved
in the viewing are brilliantly vivid.'
GUARDIAN

'[A] smart, shifting tale ... Barker is one of the
great chroniclers of the information age ...
Powerful ... a writer
in a class of her own
... A work of coruscating intelligence,
of deep humanity.'
OBSERVER

'Life-affirming **hilarity** – Evelyn Waugh on ecstasy.'
NELL ZINK

'What an audacious writer Nicola Barker is **... Punchy stuff ...** There is so much jouissance in Barker's writing.'
EVENING STANDARD

'Nicola Barker is British fiction's brightest outlier, a word-loving experimentalist whose gleeful bucking of narrative and typography most recently won her the Goldsmiths Prize ... **A madly brilliant little book ...** **I loved it.'**
DAILY MAIL

'A bracing, **brilliantly bonkers comic novel** ... This is freewheeling fiction that delights in the visual (in structure, fonts and typography) as well as in embracing language ... A sunny book.'
SUNDAY TIMES